Best wishes for health

[illegible signature]

Isaam, Mark thinking about your health. Read and Enjoy take care of the one body you are given. Mark Sept. 03.

Keeping aBreast:

Ways to PREVENT Breast Cancer

Khalid Mahmud, M.D., F.A.C.P.

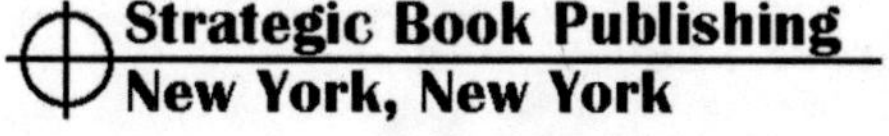

Strategic Book Publishing
An imprint of AEG Publishing Group
845 Third Avenue, 6th Floor – 6016
New York, NY 10022
http://www.strategicbookpublishing.com

ISBN: 978-1-60693-313-8, 1-60693-313-2
Printed in the United States of America
Book Design: Bruce Salender

Dedication

This book is dedicated to my mother, who instilled in me the desire and determination to become a physician; to my sisters for their boundless love; and to my wife, whose wisdom, love and support have guided me through most critical decisions in life.

Acknowledgments

I am thankful to my wife, Marilyn, for her thoughts and insight into women's issues and for her valuable comments on my first attempt at writing this book. Thanks to James McKenna, M.D., F.A.C.P. for making useful comments and for writing the foreword. Thanks to Terry Labandz for her efficient and precise editing.

I would especially like to thank my son, Shawn, for painstakingly going through the manuscript to provide many useful linguistic and scientific comments, and for his assistance on all aspects of this book.

Foreword

As a hematologist-oncologist who practiced for nearly forty years, I read *Keeping aBreast* with considerable interest. Although the book is targeted primarily at women, it is a book that health care professionals should find extremely valuable as a source of information. This is especially true for oncologists, primary-care physicians, gynecologists and nurse practitioners.

The book provides many useful tips on how to prevent breast cancer without the use of drugs, relying instead on the role of nutrition, supplements and natural hormones. Using many scientific references, the author clarifies the differences between progesterone and progestin (the former being beneficial to a woman's heart and bone health and preventive against breast cancer, while the latter is detrimental). He does the same for many other hormones that affect the quality of women's lives.

The author's explanation of the complicated hormonal changes, that occur as a woman ages, are excellent. His recommendations as to how to deal with these changes in a natural way are informative and proactive. The illustrations are masterful, cleverly done and very informative.

This book is an excellent reference for anyone involved in women's health issues.

James L. McKenna, M.D., F.A.C.P.

Contents

Contents

Introduction

A book on breast cancer prevention by a hematologist-oncologist? Why?

My struggle with my specialty of hematology-oncology began soon after I entered medical practice. I was in my early 30s, board certified in Internal Medicine and an elected fellow of the American College of Physicians (FACP), the only one from my group of residents at the Minneapolis VA to have received this title. And now, I had worked hard and completed my boards in Hematology, one of the first in the country to get this certification.

I had a sense of excitement and anticipation; everything in hematology was at my finger tips, and I was confident and happy to be practicing this specialty. Physicians in the hospital would send me consultations such as patients with leukemia and other types of cancer. I got busy in private practice, reaping its intellectual and financial rewards.

It did not occur to me that my exuberance for this specialty could be a transient state of mind. It was about to change, and begin to fade.

One morning, I was paged and asked to see a young woman who had come into the hospital with abnormal blood counts and bone marrow. I took one look at the bone marrow and knew that it was acute promyelocytic leukemia. We had seen a few cases of this type of leukemia during our hematology training; each one had died within a few weeks. These particular leukemia cells made a patient's blood clot inside the blood vessels, and in doing so exhausted the supply of normal clotting factors. The end result was uncontrollable bleeding, and death in a few weeks.

Walking towards the patient's room, I knew I had my work cut out for me. The run-of-the-mill treatment we had used previously had failed every time. It would be senseless to try it over and over again. I would have to hit these leukemic cells hard and quick, before they used up all her clotting factors. Before I reached the patient's room, I thought about using Daunomycin, the fast acting 'chemo' that had just become available, although I had not yet heard of any one using it in this particular type of leukemia.

The patient, Mary Jane (fictitious name), was 20 years old, tall, with large brown eyes, an extremely beautiful student from the University of Minnesota. She listened carefully as I detailed our findings, the diagnosis and my plan of action. She asked questions, but, as I recall, not too many. She agreed with the plan and wanted to proceed. Then she looked at me with an expression which is hard to describe. Perhaps, it was a mixture of hope, fear, trust and helplessness. As I left the room, I was deeply affected and saddened by the fact that she had such a terrible form of leukemia. She was my youngest patient with cancer.

The 'chemo' was no piece of cake, by any stretch of the imagination. Mary Jane couldn't eat, became sick, dehydrated and gaunt (this was before the days of potent anti-nausea medications), and began to lose her hair in huge clumps. She had to be supported by all possible means: infection protection measures, intravenous fluids and nourishment, transfusions of all sorts, and antibiotics. The chemo was quickly wiping out the leukemic cells and, along with those, her good blood cells too. Our hope was that, at the end, the good cells would grow back and the bad ones stay away . . . what we call a 'remission.' They finally did. After three grueling weeks, Mary Jane was in a complete remission! There were cheers and smiles all around; the nurses, myself, the family, everyone was happy. So was Mary Jane; she was happy, relieved and thankful, walking up and down the hall holding the nurse's hand. Everything was perfect . . . for now.

Everything that is, except one. During the whole ordeal, Mary Jane's boyfriend disappeared, quietly, without saying a word. Mary Jane was heart broken. Everyone felt badly for her; but, the bottom line was that she was alive.

Mary Jane went back to the U. She wanted to study hard and graduate from college. She joined the volley ball team, even found a new boyfriend. While in remission she felt normal, so she acted normal. She did the usual things like parties, going to movies, studying hard for exams, family gatherings, and made plans for the future with her new boyfriend. I saw her now and then, and looked at her blood slide (always with my fingers crossed) hoping and praying that she would stay in remission, somehow forever.

Meanwhile, I passed my boards in Oncology and developed a following of many cancer patients, whom I saw in my new clinic. They were of all kinds: some were curable, some quickly fatal, others who would go into remissions for variable lengths of time. In the beginning they would be cases like “carcinoma of the stomach,” “small cell lung cancer,” “large cell lymphoma,” “stage 2 cancer of the breast,” and so on. With time, they would change to: George, Tina, Tom or Mary. I would begin to share in their lives. They were changing from simply patients to more like friends.

I was devastated the day I found Mary Jane was out of remission. She had been healthy for more than two years and, I believe, was the longest surviving acute promyelocytic leukemia patient in the city at the time. But that thought did not console me. I had to put her through another course of debilitating chemo. She suffered through it just like the first time, with a lot of supportive care, finger crossing, and hand holding. Again, at the end of three weeks, she somehow emerged with a complete remission . . . bold, bald, sitting up straight at the edge of the hospital bed, smiling, still beautiful!

The fact that she was missing so much college, and that her second boyfriend had also disappeared, did not seem to matter too much. We were all happy that she was alive, in remission and gaining strength. There could be better days ahead.

And there were, around 600 more days, some good, some not so good. Then the moment that I had feared and had known would arrive, came calling. She had suffered a recurrence—a bad one, and this time I couldn’t get her into remission. I tried everything in the book, every possible trick in my bag, nothing worked. Finally, I contacted the leading bone marrow transplant center in Seattle, sat down with Mary Jane and her family, and presented it as the best available option. They thought about it, made a few calls, packed their bags and headed off to Seattle. Then I prayed for another remission.

Mary Jane never came back. The bone marrow transplant rejected, multiple infections developed; she fought gallantly, I am told, but in the end, lost.

Mary Jane’s picture has always remained in my mind’s eye, next to a question: “Why?” Why do things like this have to happen? Is there a way to prevent cancer?

My professional career moved on. I became the Medical Director of Oncology at my medical center. Many patients with all types of cancers came to see me. Some died right away, others were cured, yet others went into remission for variable lengths of time. As I followed those in remission, it became more and more difficult to maintain a strict doctor-patient relationship. I found myself attached to them. When and if they died, a little part of me died with them. "Duration of complete remission," "Prolongation of Survival," the usual oncology jargon, meant less and less with time. Mary Jane's story kept on repeating. Maria, the 40 year old from Argentina with cancer of the ovary, John, the gas station owner with the four year old daughter who always gave me a hug, Rosie (all fictitious names) the forty some-thing who, I thought, I had cured of lung cancer, but who secretly continued to smoke and developed a second lung cancer 10 years later, and many others.

My practice was successful and I was financially secure, but deep inside I was restless. I started a van service to treat the sicker cancer patients in their homes, and a 'cancer link program' in rural areas to give chemo to patients in their own hometowns, so they wouldn't have to travel to the big city, and be sick on their way back home. Yet, I remained troubled; troubled with losing my friend-patients and troubled with the fact that overall cancer statistics had not changed appreciably over the years in spite of all of our new therapies. I was burdened with the suspicion that we could not adequately assess the real value of time that we added to our patient's lives, and bothered by the wastefulness of American medicine, which was number one in the world on spending, but 20th on life expectancy, while providing no coverage for 1/6th of its citizens. America was spending 25% of its health care dollars during the last six months of life— some $300 billion a year to finance every conceivable treatment for every possible condition— without adding an iota to quality of life! America was doing nothing to correct problems early. We were not spending anything on prevention.

Such thoughts and other life events finally brought me to Anti-Aging Medicine, a new specialty that I practice now, a specialty that focuses on prevention. It is a specialty that tackles the mechanisms of aging and age-related diseases, in individualized patients, to create vigor, vitality and quality of life.

As I have practiced Anti-Aging Medicine, and seen predominantly female patients, my oncology background has made me increasingly conscious of the lack of preventive measures in the practice of medicine to stop breast cancer. Women follow the usual doctor's recommendations, do an occasional self exam and get a now-and-then mammogram. There is never a question by the patient, or a suggestion by the doctor, on how to prevent breast cancer. It is a disease that affects one out of eight American women, the disease most women dread. It can disfigure, mutilate and scar womanhood, and its therapy often leads to prolonged or permanent impairment in function and quality of life. Yet there is no concentrated medical effort to prevent it.

America does not lack breast cancer awareness. Numerous breast cancer groups exist in every city. The Susan G. Komen Breast Cancer Foundation has raised $750 million and spent hundreds of millions on research. The National Institute of Health and the pharmaceutical industry spend even more. However, the emphasis is on treatment, the "cure," with hundreds of new chemo and bio-therapy protocols every year, and, perhaps, a little on "early detection"- self exams and mammograms; but, none on breast cancer prevention.

The American Society of Clinical Oncology (ASCO) is the leading cancer research and education body in the world. Approximately 3,000 research abstracts are submitted to its meeting every year[1,2]. I looked at the abstract books for the last 2 years. There were about 5 abstracts related to breast cancer prevention (0.15%) each year, and those mainly focused on the use of pharmaceuticals.

Why is it, that mainstream medicine is silent on breast cancer prevention? Perhaps because:

- We physicians are primarily trained to diagnose and treat disease, with little emphasis on prevention.
- Medicare and other insurers pay us very little for prevention. Most reimbursement is based on diagnosis and treatment of disease, with specific billing codes.
- The pharmaceutical industry, which has a very significant influence on the practice of medicine, is focused on

creating and marketing cancer treatment drugs, rather than on ways to prevent it. This fact is obvious in the ASCO figures mentioned above.

The current state of American medicine does not imply a lack of information on the prevention of breast cancer. On the contrary, there are numerous scientific publications that provide insight into many useful modalities and strategies that can help reduce breast cancer. I have assembled such modalities to create a breast cancer prevention guideline for my own patients. It is based on a critical review of an extensive body of literature, and consists of simple and natural measures, things to take, things to do, with little or no use of pharmaceuticals.

My dream is to share this information with all women and their doctors with the hope that we can cut down the occurrence of this horrible disease.

How to Read This Book

My main goal in writing this book is to help reduce the occurrence—or at least delay the onset—of breast cancer in women. I would like to see the day when only one out of 12 or16, rather than one out of 8 women (the current American rate), develop this disease. Yes, we physicians have been advising women to perform self exams and get routine mammograms. But that is not prevention. It is only early detection. And it has made no significant difference in the incidence of breast cancer.

The greatest strides in health care were made when prevention became available, stopping the infectious scourges of the 19th and 20th century, such as plague, influenza and small pox – diseases which had obliterated huge sections of the world's population. More recently, lung cancer has shown signs of slowing down in the United States because of smoking cessation, a preventive measure, rather than from any breakthrough, surgical advance, or magical new chemotherapy protocol.

Producing an educational guide to prevent breast cancer will certainly be helpful to women who read it, but it may not have far reaching impact unless physicians become involved in the process. To provide credibility and authenticity, particularly for physicians, I have included references to extensive scientific work that backs the advice and measures presented herein. I have simplified complicated concepts by using lay-person language and explanatory illustrations wherever possible. As you go through the chapters in order, these concepts will become increasingly clear. At the end, you will have a real understanding of breast cancer: what starts it, what makes it grow or spread, and what makes it retreat or destruct. It is this knowledge that will be your best defense against breast cancer, and not the exclusive, ongoing and tiresome dependence on our surgical, radiological and chemotherapeutic interventions.

The book is divided into four sections. The first, the shortest section, deals with what initiates a breast cancer and how to try to stop such initiation. The second section is about promotion of breast cancer, that is, its growth once it has started. It is a discussion of the factors that promote this growth and spread. The third and the largest section deals with things that inhibit this growth, things we can use to cut down on the rate of breast cancer, or at least delay its occurrence. The fourth section consists of summary guidelines created to suit different women of different ages and risk factors, so they have a specific course to adopt and follow. Once you have read the book, you can refer only to the guideline that pertains to your needs, or look up any other chapter to refresh your knowledge on different items and factors discussed in the book.

As a physician specialized in multiple disciplines, including cancer and anti-aging medicine, with more than 30 years of clinical experience, and an understanding of how to judge medical research, I am confident that the suggestions and guidelines presented in this book, if followed, will significantly decrease the risk of this much dreaded disease in women.

Enjoy reading, learn and take action. "Know your enemy as you know yourself and you will win every battle."— Old Chinese proverb.

Note to the Reader

Please note that the information presented in this book and the guidelines developed at the end are only educational in purpose. They do not take into account your own unique medical history and clinical condition known to your personal physician. Please consult your physician before following any of the suggestions herein.

- Section 1 -
Initiation of Breast Cancer

Chapter 1
First Things First: How does a breast cancer cell start?

The Initiation

When oncologists talk about the life cycle of cancer they divide it into 3 stages: initiation, promotion and progression. ***Initiation*** is when a normal cell becomes abnormal and can divide uncontrollably and permanently.

What is it that can turn a normal breast cell into a cancer cell? Getting a handle on this is going to allow us to understand ways to minimize the process of initiation and reduce the chance of breast cancer.

Breast cancer usually develops in the cells that line the milk ducts or in the cells that form the glands which drain into the milk ducts. An essential event that has to occur is some sort of an assault on the DNA, located in the nucleus of the cell. DNA, the biological version of a computer code contained in a hundred thousand genes, is the master controller of all cellular functions. In this process (an assault on the DNA) certain genes called ***'oncogenes'*** (tumor promoting genes) may become activated, or certain ***tumor suppressor genes*** may become impaired, thus stimulating the growth of cells and making them grow uncontrollably. Thankfully there are ***DNA repair enzymes*** that move up and down the DNA molecule, like a highway repair crew, and effectively repair all such DNA damage. If this damage is not completely repaired (which happens occasionally) and the damaged cell manages to divide, this is the beginning of a cancer. Even then, our immune system, particularly the ***Natural Killer (NK) cells***, which are on constant patrol within our bodies, spot these young cancer cells as foreign invaders, attack them with lethal enzymes and destroy them. It is rare that a cell gone bad survives to become a full-fledged cancer. Our defense system has amazing capacity.

Multiple factors lead to initiation of cancer in the breast. The following seem to be the most important.

Free Radicals

Free radicals are molecules that have lost a small negative charge called an ***electron***. Because electrons like to live in pairs, a molecule with a lone electron gets very restless or ***reactive***. It tries to steal an electron from other molecules in the neighborhood. Think of a single guy in a bar late at night, trying to pair up with someone else's girlfriend. It can be quite troublesome. These free radicals attack all sorts of molecules in the cell, including enzymes, important proteins, cell wall, even the DNA. Anti-oxidants that naturally exist in our cells and those that we consume mop up and neutralize these free radicals. However, the onslaught continues. Our DNA can take several thousand hits from such free radicals every day. Only once in a while a cell with damaged DNA escapes our defense system and becomes a cancer.

In the breast, there is an unappreciated mechanism for the formation of free radicals. It is the fluid that accumulates and gets pent up in the milk glands and ducts. Studies have shown that this fluid eventually breaks down and forms free radicals[3, 4]. Right next to this fluid are the cells lining the ducts and glands (alveoli), which must bear the brunt of these radicals (see fig 1). These are the cells that commonly become malignant in the breast. "***Ductal cancer***" is the most common type of breast cancer.

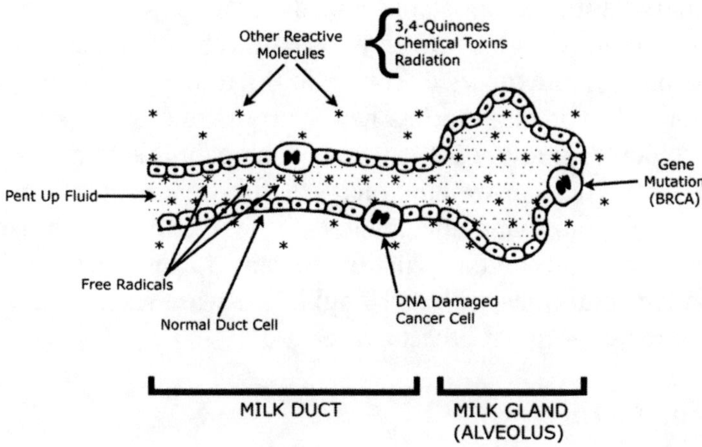

Fig 1. Breast Cancer Initiation

Studies from 30 different countries[5] have proven that the breast cancer rate is lower in women who breast feed their babies. However, the mechanism involved in this protection has not been well explained and remains somewhat of a mystery. The most logical explanation — in my mind — is that breast feeding cleanses the milk ducts; it removes the free radicals. Breast feeding increases the level of the hormone ***oxytocin,*** which not only contracts duct muscles to propel the fluid but also has additional anti-cancer actions that I will explain later. In this regard, it is of interest to mention that the Tanka fisherwomen of Hong Kong breast feed their babies only on one side. When they develop breast cancer, 8 out of 10 times it is in the unused side.

There are other ways in which free radicals and reactive molecules are generated in the breast that may be important in the process of initiation. For example, estrogen, through metabolism, can change into a substance called ***3, 4-quinone,*** which can create free radicals[6]. The exact role of these substances in the initiation of breast cancer is unknown. It has been argued that an average pre-menopausal breast does not contain enough estrogen to generate sufficient *3, 4-quinone* to cause significant damage.

Similarly, radiation can create a type of radical called ***hydroxyl (OH) free radical.*** Some people have argued that mammograms can contribute to the causation of breast cancer. However, the amount of radiation administered and the free radicals generated by a mammogram would be much too small to be of concern. As a rule, a mammogram exposes a woman to 0.1 to 0.2 rad (a measure of radiation). A woman who has had yearly mammograms for 20 years has received a total of 2 to 4 rads. Compare this to a dose of 3,000 to 4,000 rads a woman receives for treatment of breast cancer and mammograms appear pretty safe. On the other hand, women who have received radiation therapy to the chest during childhood for conditions such as Hodgkin's disease seem to have a higher risk for subsequent breast cancer.

Chemical Toxins

Hundreds of chemical toxins constantly enter our bodies, from the environment, food and water. There are many names for these, such as aromatic amines, aromatic hydrocarbons, heterocyclic amines, nitroso compounds, dioxins and the like. Many of these are present in pesticides, solvents, plastic, well cooked or charred meat, industry discharge, etc. Most of these toxins are organic compounds, meaning that they are soluble in fat rather than water, and therefore tend to accumulate in the body fat, such as in the breast. As long as they are stored, they are essentially harmless. It is only when the body tries to get rid of them that they become activated and begin to cause damage. Let me explain how.

The body removes harmful toxins in two stages. First, the so called ***"phase 1 enzymes,"*** also known as P 450 enzymes, change them into intermediate metabolites. These intermediate metabolites are extremely ***reactive,*** like free radicals; they cause DNA damage and damage to other molecules. These reactive molecules have to be removed immediately, before they can cause harm. That is the job of the ***"phase II enzymes."*** The phase II enzymes quickly convert them into harmless entities that can be easily excreted from the body, via the intestinal or urinary tracts. These detoxifying enzymes can be impaired with age, poor health, alcohol and certain pharmaceuticals.

It is of interest to note here that ***Premarin***, the horse derived estrogen given to women for decades, is not identical to human estrogen; it actually inactivates one of these important phase II enzymes, the ***glutathione S transferase***[7]! Could this account for some of the increase in breast cancer among women who received Premarin based HRT? I believe it is quite likely to be the case.

Gene abnormalities

There are many gene abnormalities (***mutations***) that lead to cancer. With greater understanding of the human genome and the increasing ease with which these abnormalities can be detected, the role of genes in cancer is unfolding every day. Many of these gene abnormalities are induced by chemicals such as those mentioned above, some are caused by viruses, while other cancer causing gene abnormalities are inherited.

The most well known hereditary mutations pertinent to breast cancer are those of the genes called ***BRCA 1*** and ***BRCA II***. When working normally, these genes are "***cancer suppressor genes***." They prevent normal cells from becoming cancerous.[8] Women who inherit either of these gene abnormalities have a 70% chance of developing breast cancer by age 70. Those with BRCA 1 mutations have an additional 40% chance of cancer of the ovary by the same age. Overall these gene abnormalities are responsible for only 5% to 10% of all breast cancers in women.

Other genetic factors seem to increase the risk of breast cancer. For instance, women whose mothers or paternal grandmothers had breast cancer have an increased risk for developing this disease.

I am sure as time passes and we learn more about breast cancer, other factors will emerge that have important bearing on the initiation of breast cancer. On the other hand, fears that breast injury, coffee drinking or silicone implants cause breast cancer are without scientific basis.

Chapter 2
How to Reduce the Initiation of Breast Cancer—Nip It in the Bud

BRCA Gene Abnormalities

Currently, we cannot do much to prevent the **BRCA** gene abnormalities: it is not possible to choose your parents. But, physicians and patients can work together to improve the final outcome for those with hereditary BRCA abnormalities.

Women who have multiple family members with breast cancer should be encouraged to see a geneticist and undergo genetic screening and counseling for these abnormalities. If they turn out to be positive, they generally would have two options: a path of careful observation with frequent exams, mammograms and the necessary biopsies, or surgical removal of both breasts with reconstruction and implants, and possibly endoscopic removal of the ovaries.

A woman's choice in this situation is not easy. It needs candid, and often multiple, discussions with the patient and her family. Second opinions are often necessary, which can be taxing and emotionally draining. The patient and the family should be given enough time and provided with as much explanation as necessary to make a decision with which she can be content. Some women are comfortable with a careful "wait-and-watch attitude." Others are "nervous wrecks," they cannot sleep, get depressed or panic; their quality of life is significantly impaired. They may want to have both their breasts and ovaries removed, and desire implants, which I think is OK. After all, there are hundreds of thousands of women who have implants for aesthetic purposes only. Why not for those with BRCA mutations?

I have seen both types of patients in my practice. I also have a patient whose mother and younger sister have breast cancer. She feels she is better off not knowing and has declined to go through BRCA testing. Meanwhile we are doing everything we can to prevent breast cancer and her GYN doctor is keeping a careful watch. Such decisions are personal and should ultimately be left to a woman's discretion. I believe physicians should explain, not push women in any one direction.

Fruits and Vegetables have been considered to reduce the risk of breast and other cancers, and epidemiological studies suggest that they do so.[9] There are several possible mechanisms for this benefit.

Fruits and vegetable are rich sources of anti-oxidants that quench free radicals.[10] They contain hundreds of ***bio-flavanoids*** (plant chemicals) that have anti-cancer properties, including the fact that they turn on the phase II enzymes,[11, 12] enzymes that rid our bodies of cancer-causing toxins. They also provide fiber that binds the toxins excreted into the intestine, so that these toxins are not absorbed back into the system.

In spite of the fact that some studies question the role of fruits and vegetables,[13] it is an overall consensus, world wide, that fruits and vegetables are healthy. They not only reduce the rate of cancer, but also prevent atherosclerosis and heart disease. I believe women (and men) of all ages should try to eat as many fruits and vegetables as possible, but avoid some of the high-glycemic fruits (those that raise the blood sugar the highest) such as ripe bananas and pineapple.

I routinely advise my patients to supplement with vegetable and fruit extracts, since it is difficult to eat 'five servings of fruits and vegetables each day.' Several such supplements are available as capsules or in powder form.

Excess body fat has been found to increase the risk for breast cancer by 30% to 50%.[14] There are many studies that prove this association. More body fat stores more toxins, and generates more free radicals to initiate breast cancer. In addition, excess body fat is a promoter of breast cancer growth, as we will discuss later.

Women should make every effort to keep their body fat below 25%. As we all know, our lifestyle, the food sold in supermarkets and restaurants, and our eating habits have made it nearly impossible for most of us to be lean. More than 60% of Americans are over weight; and the epidemic is growing. Ten years ago, one out of ten American women were getting breast cancer. Now it is one out of eight, and there is a suggestion that it is moving closer to one in seven!

Exposure to toxins should be minimized by all means.

One should avoid well done or fried meat as this process generates ***heterocyclic amines***.

Organic produce should be preferred to super-market fruits and vegetables to cut down on pesticides. As a rule, all food should be as simple and natural as possible. Enriching and processing almost always leads to unhealthful consequences. Solvents (such as nail polish), cooking in plastic bags, and spraying insecticides without protection should be avoided. While working with household cleansers, protective gloves should be worn.

Pent up breast duct fluid, as I have discussed before, is a source of free radicals that are damaging to the DNA of the cells of breast ducts, the site where most breast cancers develop.

In this regard, it is important to talk about the hormone ***oxytocin***. Oxytocin is secreted by the pituitary gland in response to a baby's cry or during suckling; it causes contraction of the breast ducts to propel the milk. The process naturally cleans the ducts of any pent up fluid so that free radicals do not accumulate. In addition, oxytocin has a direct anti-cancer effect that will be discussed in a later chapter.

This is why populations where women breast feed have very little breast cancer. I was born in Pakistan many years ago. There was no such thing as baby formulas. My mother breast fed me for two years and so did all of the other women in the family and the neighborhood for their children. I never heard of any one of those women getting breast cancer. Women should breast feed their babies as long as possible. It does not help to fool Mother Nature.

Dr. T.G. Murrell from the University of Adelaide, Australia, has preached the use of breast and nipple massage to prevent breast cancer.[4, 15] Studies have shown that a 10-minute mechanical stimulation of the breasts in normal women increases the blood oxytocin level by up to 100%.[16] Oxytocin not only propels the fluid in the breast ducts, but is also inhibitory to cancer cells. It makes perfect sense for women to engage in this maneuver on a regular basis. It is free, harmless, and has the potential of preventing breast cancers.

Although preventing initiation of breast cancer is important, and all efforts should be made to stop this process, inhibition of promotion, the second phase, seems to be more important for all practical purposes. It is so because by the time most women start thinking about breast cancer (usually in their late thirties or forties), those destined to get one have already 'initiated' it in one of their breasts. The rest of this book is mainly a discussion of factors that promote or inhibit the promotion of breast cancer, and how to influence these factors to diminish the impact of this disease.

- Section 2 -
Promotion of Breast Cancer

Chapter 3
Promotion: What makes a tiny cancer grow after it has been initiated?

Most people, even many doctors, don't know how long it takes a cancer cell to grow to be a full-fledged tumor. The general impression is that cancer just shows up, or maybe takes a few months to a year to develop. The reality is that from the time of initiation of a cancer cell to its diagnosis as a cancer, between fifteen to twenty years have elapsed. It is true that some cancers grow faster, particularly leukemias, and others much more slowly, such as prostate cancer. But for most cancers this time period is 15-20 years.

After a cancer cell has been initiated, its growth into a tumor depends on its doubling time. That is, the time taken for 1 tumor cell to turn in to 2, 2 to 4, 4 to 8, and so forth. The doubling time of many cancers is quite slow and can range from many months to years.[17] Although the cells divide faster, many are lost or killed by our natural killer (NK) cells and other factors that inhibit their growth, so the net doubling time of the tumors is much slower. The average doubling time of breast cancer has been found to be around six months.[18] A cancer cell has to go through 20 doublings to become the size of one millimeter, another 10 doublings to attain the size of one centimeter, and another 10 doublings to reach a generally fatal size of 10 cm. The usual size of a breast cancer upon diagnosis is around 2 centimeters, although in certain parts of the country it may be larger, and in 3rd world countries, larger still.

It may be a surprise to realize that a woman diagnosed with breast cancer at age 45 actually started out with the first cancer cell at around age 27. Although most breast cancer occurs in post-menopausal women (80%), it frequently starts before menopause.

During its long period of latency, the tiny breast cancer is influenced by many factors. Some of these are ***promoters*** and some ***inhibitors*** of growth. If we recognize and understand these factors, we can influence or change them, and by doing so, slow down the process of growth.

We can, thus, prevent or delay the appearance of breast cancer (Fig 2).

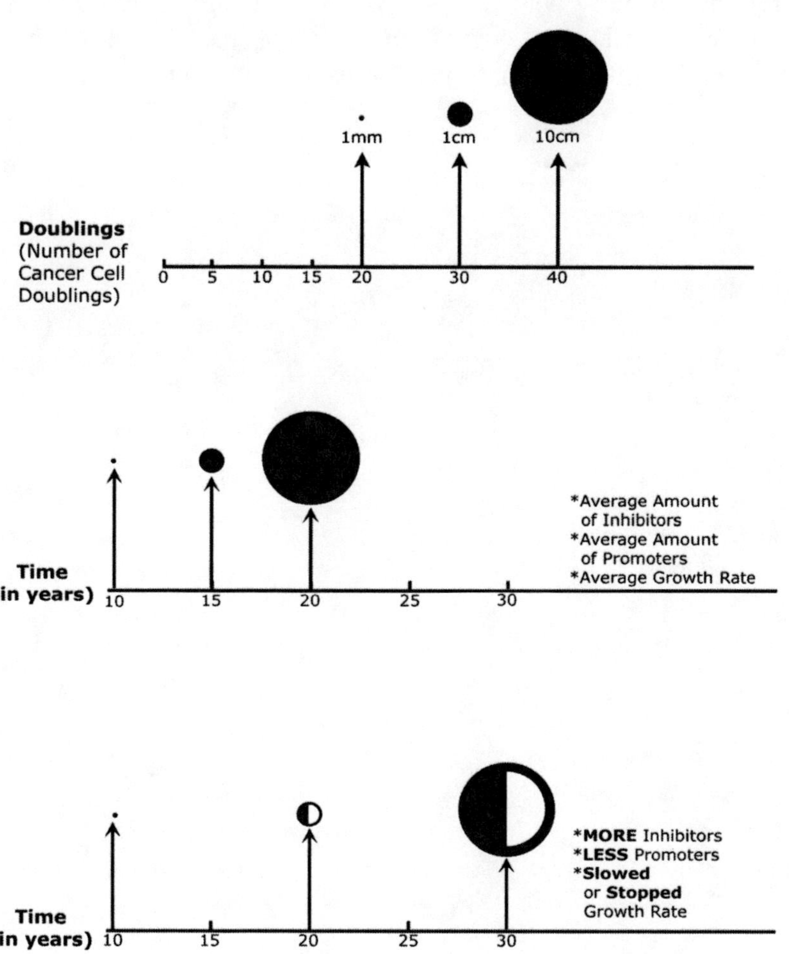

Fig. 2—Breast Cancer Growth and Promotion Timelines and the Concept of Slowing or Stopping Growth.

Many things promote breast cancer, such as free radicals, certain (strong) estrogens, insulin, alcohol, etc. Others inhibit it.

Examples of these are: plant derivatives, certain hormones, some vitamins, foods, exercise, etc. The remainder of this book is a detailed discussion of these factors. First we will discuss the promoters of breast cancer, then the inhibitors. We will identify ways to blunt or diminish the promoters and strengthen the inhibitors to our advantage. At the end, the entire discussion will be summarized into a guideline for the prevention of breast cancer— the guideline that I use for my own patients.

Chapter 4
Estrogens that can promote breast cancer—the friends who can hurt

Estrogen is the essence of womanhood. It creates fullness in the breasts, curves in the body, and glow in the skin. It is responsible for a woman's mindset, emotions and sensuality. Estrogen is essential for sexual and reproductive function. It lubricates the vagina. During the menstrual cycle, estrogen and progesterone prepare the womb for implantation of an embryo. However, sex and reproduction are not the only reasons why estrogen exists. It promotes health in many different ways; in fact, it has an effect on almost every tissue in the body.

The protective effects of estrogen on the heart have been documented by many scientific studies over the years. These benefits were recently detailed by Dr. Michael Mendelsohn (Tufts University Molecular Cardiology Research Institute) in an excellent review in the American Journal of Cardiology.[19] Estrogen dilates or opens the coronary arteries, prevents damage to the lining of blood vessels, increases good cholesterol (HDL), decreases triglycerides, and fights atherosclerosis. In my 30 years of medical practice, I have seen many men in their early forties who came to the ER with a heart attack, but almost never a woman at that age.

Brain and bone, two vital structures in the body, are heavily dependent on estrogen for their integrity. Estrogen enhances memory by growing nerve connections in the memory centers of the brain; it protects nerve cells against free radicals and from Beta-amyloid protein that causes Alzheimer's disease.[20]

Almost 40% of the women in our nursing homes are there because they broke a bone…usually a hip. Estrogen, progesterone and testosterone all strengthen the bone, prevent osteoporosis and reduce the chance of these fractures.

In short, estrogen not only creates what some famous gynecologists call "woman-ness," but is essential for the health and vitality of a woman's entire body and mind.

Yet, where there are roses, there can be thorns! Some

estrogens, under certain circumstances, stimulate the growth of breast cancer. Let us see how.

A woman's body produces three estrogens: ***estrone, estradiol and estriol***. Estradiol is further metabolized into 2 compounds: ***2-hydroxyestrone*** and ***16 alpha-hydroxyestrone.*** Some estrogens can be bad under certain circumstances and promote breast cancer. Others have been called good estrogens because they slow or inhibit the growth of breast cancer. Let us see how some estrogens can be "bad."

Estrone and estradiol are strong estrogens. Despite their benefits, they stimulate the growth of normal breast cells as well as breast cancer cells. Many breast cancer cells, especially those in post-menopausal women, have ***estrogen receptors (ER)***, which use estradiol and estrone to fuel their growth (fig 3).

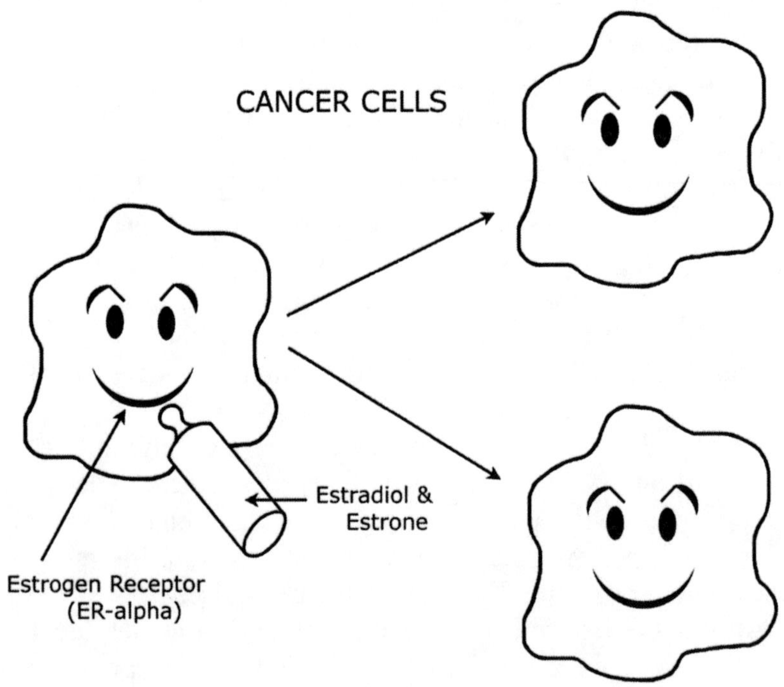

Breast Cancer Promotion by Estradiol (E2) and Estrone (E1)

Fig. 3

It is well known that women who had early menarche or late menopause tend to have more breast cancer. Why is that so? The reason is that these strong estrogens rise to high levels during parts of the menstrual cycle; so the more menstrual cycles a woman has in her lifetime, the more exposure her breasts have had to these strong estrogens. If that woman has cancer cells in her breast, those cells could be stimulated by these estrogens. It has also been suggested that estrogen dominant women (those with high estrogen and low progesterone levels) are at a higher risk for breast cancer, because they lack the protection provided by progesterone against estrogen. I will discuss the protective role of progesterone in a later chapter.

Does that mean giving estrogen to menopausal women is a bad idea? Not necessarily so. Let me explain why.

Menopausal women with breast cancer have higher blood and urine levels of estrogen compared to their normal cohorts,[21] but pre-menopausal breast cancer patients do not show such a clear cut difference. In fact, some studies suggest that they may even have less estrogen in their urine.[22]

When women are young, all estrogen is made in the ovaries. As they age, their ovaries slow down and the body's fat cells begin to make estrogen. An enzyme called ***aromatase*** in the fat cells converts testosterone into estrogen. By the time women are in menopause, their ovaries are non-functional, and most estrogen is manufactured in the fat cells, that is, in the buttocks, thighs and breasts. The blood level of estrogen is then 5 to 15 times less than what it had been before menopause. It is just a reflection of how much estrogen is being produced in the fatty tissue.

Studies have shown that the breast tissue of women with breast cancer has 10 to 50 times the concentration of estrogens than what is in their blood.[23, 24, 25] The breast tissue in such women shows increased aromatase, which is particularly concentrated around the tumor,[26] producing estrogen in high concentration and fueling the growth of the tumor. Because estrogen can seep out from the site of its formation into the blood, it is easy to understand why the blood (and urine) level of estrogen is higher in these post-menopausal women with breast cancer. On the other hand, pre-menopausal women have much higher blood levels of estrogen to begin with. If there is a cancer in the breast, that would have little or minimal effect on this already-high blood level. A dime added to a dime in your pocket can double your money, but won't make much difference if you already had a dollar in your pocket.

Therefore, giving small amounts of estrogen (amounts that do not cause breast tenderness) to post-menopausal women would increase their blood estrogen level somewhat, but would have no significant effect on breast estrogen level, which is already much higher than in the blood. It would be like a drop in the bucket, and would therefore not increase the risk of breast cancer. Many studies suggest that this is the case.

The recent large Women's Health Initiative (WHI) study in America[27] and Women's Health in the Lund Area (WHILA) study in Sweden[28] revealed that menopausal women receiving Premarin and Provera (artificial, synthetic hormones) have a higher occurrence of breast cancer. However, women who received estrogen alone had no such effect.

One of the largest HRT studies, of 23,000 Swiss women, most of whom took estradiol or estriol (unlike the popular American combination of Premarin and Provera) showed that there was a 28% decrease in death from breast cancer.[29]

An important study of 319 women took place at M.D. Anderson Cancer Center, Houston, and was reported in the Journal of Clinical Oncology.[30] These women had a localized breast cancer removed. Two years later, 39 of these women were started on estrogen. After six years, only one woman developed a new breast cancer. On the other hand 14 women in the control group (those who did not take estrogen) developed new or recurrent breast cancer. In other words, some increase in the blood level of estrogen had no effect on the reoccurrence of breast cancer. In fact, it seemed to prevent it.

Another study looked at menopausal women who had had a localized breast cancer. After 5 years of estrogen therapy 3.6% of the women developed new breast cancer compared with 13.5% in the group who did not take estrogen .[31]

What all of these studies demonstrate is the fact that it is not the estrogen therapy in post-menopausal women that promotes breast cancer, but the estrogen produced in the breast itself, and especially around an existing cancer, that fuels this growth (fig 4).

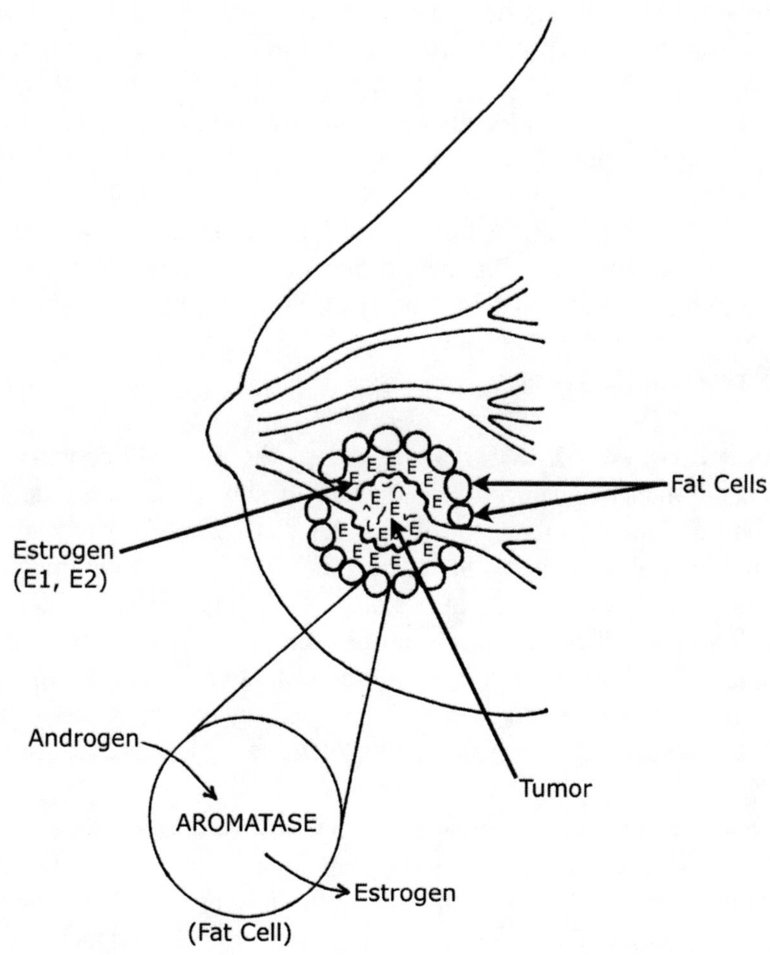

Fig 4—Breast fat cells producing estrogen to fuel cancer growth.

Unfortunately, the Women's Health Initiative (WHI) Premarin plus Provera study results have scared doctors and women into stopping all estrogen therapy in women. The side effects seen in this study can be attributed to the use of ***artificial and synthetic hormones***, which are foreign to the human body. These substances are not the hormones that exist in a woman's body. Real hormones create health rather than disease. These real ***natural bio-identical*** hormones have been available for years, but, unfortunately are ignored. If artificial substances cause harm to your health, you cannot say that natural hormones would do the same. If you drank water from a well all your life, then it dried up when you were 50 and you received soda pop instead for the next 15 years — leading to diabetes — you could not conclude that drinking water would have caused diabetes. Yet this is exactly what is being promulgated.

The sad part of all of this is that baby boomers, now entering menopause, with their increasing heart attacks, hip fractures and Alzheimer's disease, will not only suffer more, but also severely burden the Medicare system — a system already destined for bankruptcy in 15 years.

16 alpha-hydroxyestrone is one of the metabolites (product of metabolism) of estradiol. It has been shown to stimulate the growth of breast cancer.[32, 33] A low fat diet seems to decrease the formation of this harmful estrogen,[34] while high animal fat consumption seems to increase it. Vegetables and certain supplements reduce the formation of this "bad" estrogen. In a later chapter, I will discuss ways to decrease the formation of this harmful estrogen and to increase estrogen conversion into metabolites that are beneficial and protective against breast cancer.

Xenoestrogens is a term applied to many toxins (mostly organic chlorines) released into the environment by many industries and added to our food by the farming and food industries. They tend to accumulate in the body fat such as the breast tissue, and have a role in the initiation as well as in the promotion of breast cancer.[35] These xenoestrogens are directly toxic to DNA and act as estrogens by attaching to the estrogen receptors on the cells. They have contributed to the rising rate of breast cancer in western countries. It has been said that Israel was able to reduce the rate of breast cancer by banning organochlorine pesticides in 1976. You can cut down your exposure to these toxins by following these simple recommendations:

- Avoid contaminated fish (dioxins). Most farmed fish is contaminated. Alaskan wild salmon seems to have the least contamination

- Avoid non-organic produce, which contains pesticide residue
- Do not use plastic containers for food. Especially do no heat food in plastic bags or containers
- Avoid herbicides and insecticides
- Avoid bleached paper such as coffee filters, tissue paper, napkins, etc; EPA has estimated that lifetime use of coffee filters increases the risk of exposure to dioxins to unacceptable levels
- Avoid the use of household chlorine containing bleach, or use disposable gloves and good ventilation if you have to work with such chemicals
- Try organic sanitary napkins and tampons
- Minimize use of solvents such as nail polish

To summarize, estrogens are immensely important for women and women's health, but it is important to understand them, to know how to avoid the ones that can cause harm, and how to use them to enhance women's health.

Chapter 5
Free Radicals and Cancer Promotion

In chapter one, we discussed the role of free radicals in the initiation of breast cancer.[3, 4] The fluid pent up in the breast glands and ducts breaks down over time and releases free radicals, which damage DNA, thus inducing cancer.

Free radicals not only induce cancer but also make it grow. Many studies have demonstrated their tumor promotion capacity in animal models and their inhibition by anti-oxidants.[36, 37] Free radicals seem to be able to grow cancer cells by several different mechanisms. For example, it has been shown that they damage ***p53****,* an important tumor-suppressor gene that normally prevents the division of cells with damaged DNA and protects us from many types of cancer.[38, 39] They increase ***Protein Kinase C****,* a key enzyme that stimulates the division and growth of malignant cells.[40]

Many toxins from air, food and water (pesticides, dioxins, PCBs, heterocyclic amines, etc.) accumulate in the breasts fatty tissue. These are converted into reactive compounds, which, like free radicals, induce and promote growth of cancer cells.

Smoking is a cause of excessive free radical formation in the body. Smokers' milk duct fluid often turns dark in color. A recent study in Japan found that women who smoked had a higher than normal incidence of breast cancer.[41]

As I mentioned in chapter 2, regular breast and nipple stimulation has been proposed as a means to get rid of pent up secretions in the breast ducts. I believe this practice should be added to regular breast self examination. It makes a great deal of theoretical sense.

Intake of anti-oxidants from supplements, fruits and vegetables should be increased to curtail free radical induced initiation and promotion of cancer. I will discuss the role of anti-oxidants such as vitamin E, selenium and fruits and vegetables in chapters 20, 21 and 22, in more detail.

Smoking should be avoided as it creates a great deal of free radicals.

Finally, chemicals in food and water should be avoided (see chapter 4), not just for breast cancer prevention, but for overall health.

Chapter 6
Insulin and Insulin-like Growth Factor-1 (IGF-1)

Insulin is an important hormone that controls the metabolism of carbohydrates and brings our blood sugar down when it is elevated. As we eat more and more carbohydrates and produce more and more insulin, our system finally gets tired of handling excessive carbohydrates, and we develop what is called ***Insulin Resistance***. Our insulin level rises, but is less effective in controlling the blood sugar. As it gets worse, we develop Type II diabetes. There are 18 million diabetics in the United States, and it has been estimated that one out three Americans — 95 million — have insulin resistance.

Clearly, this is not a good situation. Insulin resistance leads to many health problems, including an increased risk of breast cancer.

Insulin is a ***growth factor***, and as it rises, it tends to increase one of its relatives, ***Insulin- like Growth Factor-1 (IGF-1)*** which is normally generated in the liver by human growth hormone, and is responsible for many of the actions of growth hormone. Both of these growth factors stimulate an enzyme, ***Tyrosine Kinase***, which directly enhances the proliferation of tumor cells.[42]

Multiple researchers have demonstrated this association. A recent study reported from Vanderbilt University suggests that insulin resistance and increased IGF-1 synergistically increase the risk for breast cancer. Women with both of these abnormalities had a three fold rise in the incidence of this disease.[43]

Dr. Pamela Goodwin (Mount Sinai Hospital, Toronto) found something even worse. She recently reported, in the Journal of Clinical Oncology, that women with early stage breast cancer, who also had a high fasting insulin level, had a higher rate of metastases (cancer spread to other organs) and death compared to those whose insulin levels were normal.[44]

Although some studies have questioned the association of IGF-1 with breast cancer,[45] a ***meta-analysis*** (combined analysis of multiple studies) of 21 studies published in 2004 has confirmed this trend.[46] Insulin resistance tends to increase IGF-1, particularly free IGF-1 (not bound to proteins and free to act on cells), which stimulates the growth and division of cancer cells.

Of course, type 2 diabetes, an advanced stage of insulin resistance, leads to more breast cancer. The American Nurses Health Study, which included 116,488 female nurses, has shown this to be true.[47]

It is somewhat ironic that the U.S. Government's Food Pyramid actually contributed to this state of affairs. The now defunct pyramid was essentially based on carbohydrates. It encouraged the intake of carbohydrates. Our food industry made matters worse by adding carbohydrates at every opportunity, even when trying to limit fats. In fact, most fat free versions of popular foods have simply had fat replaced by more carbohydrates for taste. Then, to add insult to injury, our food industry introduced giant sizes for Colas, burgers, fries, shakes, and everything else.

Now, we have the rate of diabetes increasing by 50% every decade. Insulin resistance and its accompaniment, ***visceral fat*** (belly fat), are at epidemic proportions. The health consequences of this situation will be enormous. Beside an increased rate of breast cancer, there will be more hypertension, high cholesterol, heart attack, stroke and other types of cancer. Predictions are now being made that the United States life expectancy is about to decline for the first time in history.

High insulin levels and insulin resistance are partly genetic, and are partly related to one's life style. You may have a genetic tendency towards diabetes, in which case you would be less tolerant of carbohydrates and tend to have higher insulin levels compared to a person who eats the same amount of carbohydrates but has not inherited any such tendency. However, life-style (eating large amounts of refined carbohydrates and plain sugar) can override your normal genetics and give you high insulin levels and insulin resistance. You can generally spot a person with high insulin level and insulin resistance without even doing a blood test. If such person is overweight and has an apple shape (most weight in the belly and upper body), he/she is most likely insulin resistant and has a high insulin level.

I will discuss my approach toward weight loss in the final guidelines; but, a few pointers to help reduce insulin and insulin intolerance may be helpful here:

- Reduce overall carbohydrate intake. Limit it to whole grains, vegetables and minimal fruits. Omit refined carbohydrates (white bread, pasta, rice, potato) and sugar (colas, cakes, cookies, pies). If having a burger in a restaurant, try throwing away the bun and changing it into a lettuce-burger. You will develop a taste for it in a few tries. Forget the French fries.
- Start your day with a protein rich breakfast and have adequate amount of protein at every meal. If your ideal weight is 130lbs, you need at least 75 grams of protein daily, for 160lbs it will be 90gms. If you multiply your ideal wt in pounds by 0.55, it will give you the number of grams of protein you need every day. You can roughly figure out how much protein you are eating if you know that …

  One and a quarter cup of milk has 20gms of protein
  One egg-white equals 4-5gms of protein
  Half cup of cottage cheese has 15gms
  One scoop of protein powder generally has 20gms
  Six ounces of fish, chicken or turkey has 40gms, and
  A nine ounce steak has 60gms of protein.

  It also helps to look at labels to find the protein content.
- Avoid hydrogenated or partially hydrogenated fats (read labels) as they stiffen your cell membranes so insulin receptors become blunted and don't respond to insulin
- Eat slowly and always stop eating before you are full. If in a restaurant, take half of your meal home for another dinner. They always serve too much in a restaurant. Portion size is extremely important in weight management.
- Certain supplements (chromium, alpha lipoic acid) improve insulin sensitivity. Try these supplements if you are apple shaped and overweight

Frequently, losing weight and maintaining it is not an easy process. You may wish to consult a professional who focuses on weight management.

Chapter 7
Silent Inflammation Induced By Our Diet

Silent inflammation in the body is emerging as an important mechanism leading to many modern day chronic diseases including heart disease, immune disorders, Alzheimer's disease and cancer. It is not an inflammation that we can see or feel; it just eats away at our health, imperceptibly. Doctors often measure it by ordering the test ***"C-reactive Protein" or CRP***. There are other tests to measure it that are more complicated and not used in every day medical practice.

Silent inflammation is frequently related to our food and lifestyle. It occurs when there is an imbalance of hormones called ***Prostaglandins,*** which are made inside all of the body's cells rather than in glands. There are 3 important prostaglandins: ***PG-1, PG-2 and PG-3*** (names simplified for this discussion). PG-2 is inflammatory, and PG-1 and 3 are anti-inflammatory (reduce inflammation). Let us see how all this works.

There is an important fatty acid in the body called ***Arachidonic Acid*** (***AA***), which is converted, by an enzyme called ***COX-2*** into ***PG-2.*** We need this inflammatory response to fight infections and to heal wounds. We cannot live without it. On the other hand, we don't need it to be turned on continuously. Unfortunately, our diet and lifestyle has done just that. This system is constantly activated in many of us. We have silent inflammation.

The types of fats we eat and the relative amounts of carbohydrate and protein we ingest have an important bearing on the amount of inflammation generated in our bodies (see Fig 5).

Saturated fats (meat, eggs) are a direct source of ***AA*** and therefore ***PG-2***. In other words they are inflammatory in nature.

During the past several decades, as the medical establishment discouraged saturated fats, another source of AA has emerged, the ***omega-6 vegetable oils***. These omega-6 oils are first converted into ***GLA*** (***gamma linoleic acid)*** in the body, and then either into AA and PG-2 (inflammatory) or into PG-1 (anti-inflammatory). The ratio of these two prostaglandins depends on what else you have eaten with this meal. A predominantly carbohydrate meal generates insulin that shifts this ratio towards inflammation, while a protein meal produces the hormone glucagon, which tips the balance more towards an anti-inflammatory state (see Fig 5).

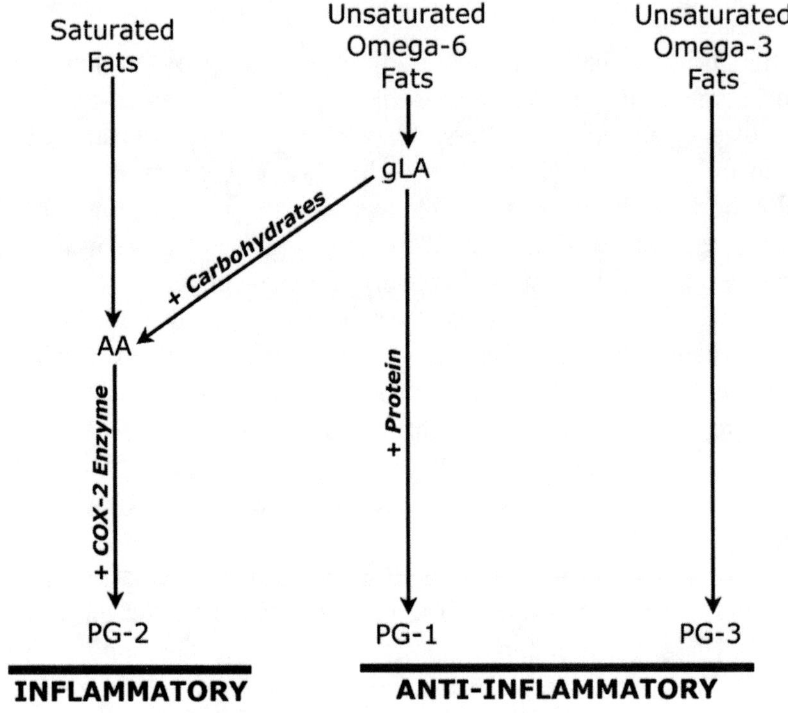

Fig. 5—How One's Diet Can Produce or Reduce Inflammation.

Dr. Barry Sear has emphasized this point in his best-selling book, "***The Zone Diet.***" It is important to eat protein at every meal, because it cuts down on the amount of silent inflammation occurring in your bodies. On the other hand, the food pyramid, which encouraged too many carbohydrates, leads to more inflammation.

Again, the pivotal enzyme creating inflammation is the COX-2. This is the enzyme that is blocked by anti-inflammatory drugs such as aspirin and ibuprofen, and the popular, but now condemned, arthritis drugs such as Celebrex and Vioxx. I will talk about these drugs later in the book.

Another important anti-inflammatory prostaglandin is ***PG-3***. It is derived from ***omega-3 fats*** in our food; mostly from deep-sea fish or fish oils, but also from flaxseed and walnuts. During our evolution, we humans used to eat a lot of omega-3 fats because they were plentiful not only in fish, but also in all types of wild game. The ratio of omega 6 to 3, in our diet, was close to1:1. Currently, this ratio is 15:1. Naturally, this has made us more prone to silent inflammation. Studies have revealed that improving this ratio (higher intake of omega-3s) can cut down the risk of many diseases including breast cancer.[48]

Silent inflammation promotes cancer in many ways:

- It promotes formation of new blood vessels which feed a tumor and help it spread
- It prevents self destruction (***apoptosis***) of cancer cells,
- It stimulates aromatase formation in the fat cells surrounding a tumor in the breast, thus making more estrogen, which, in turn fuels the growth of cancer cells. It has been shown that aromatase is directly stimulated by PG-2.[49]

A meta-analysis of multiple studies shows that reducing dietary intake of fat results in lowering of serum estrogen levels, suggesting a decrease in aromatase.[50] This may be due to the fact that decreased overall fat intake results in decreased AA and PG-2. However, part of this change may be related to less body fat producing less aromatase.

International data and case-control studies show a correlation between fat intake and breast cancer rates.[51] It is difficult to decipher the results, however, because all fats are not bad. Several experimental animal studies support the relationship between fat and breast cancer.[52] There is evidence that Omega-6 fatty acids stimulate several stages of breast cancer, while Omega-3 fatty acids seem to provide protection against it.[53]

To summarize, it makes sense to try to decrease silent inflammation in the body by dietary manipulations. One can do it by eating: less carbohydrates, more proteins, less saturated and omega 6 fats and more omega 3 fats.

Chapter 8
Excess Body Fat

Never eat more than you can lift – Miss Piggy

Americans hold the distinction of being the heaviest people in the world. Sixty percent of us are overweight and approximately 30% could be categorized as obese. Not a very pretty picture! The people who gave the world refined petroleum, the motor car, traffic lights, airplanes, computers, Windows®, the Internet, and most scientific marvels of the 20th century, are falling victim to another one of their own creations: the food industry. Our food industry, besides toxic inclusions, has given us fat . . . huge amounts of fat.

Fat, especially visceral (abdominal) fat is at the root of many ailments. Hypertension, diabetes, atherosclerosis, heart attacks, strokes, arthritis, and cancer are all related to visceral fat.

How can obesity (excess fat) lead to breast cancer? Let us look at the mechanisms (Fig 6).

As I have mentioned before, most cancer-causing toxins are fat soluble substances. They accumulate in our body fat. The more body fat, the more room for the toxins to be stored in the body. We can excrete more of these by reducing body fat and by eating fiber that binds to them once they are excreted in the intestine so they are not reabsorbed into the bloodstream.[54]

Fat cells also contain the enzyme, ***aromatase*** (discussed previously), which converts testosterone into estrogens. This is why overweight and obese women have more estrogen. The more estrogen produced in the breast tissue, the more chance of stimulating the growth of breast cancer cells

Another accompaniment of excess body fat is the excess production of insulin. As we discussed in chapter 6, increased insulin tends to increase insulin like growth factor-1 (IGF-1). Both insulin and IGF-1 are growth factors that promote the growth of breast cancer cells.

Fat produces certain substances called ***cytokines*** that are inflammatory in nature.[55] As I have explained previously, inflammation is an important cause of a whole host of chronic disease, including cancer. Most common cancers, such as those of the breast, prostate, colon and lung, are promoted by silent inflammation

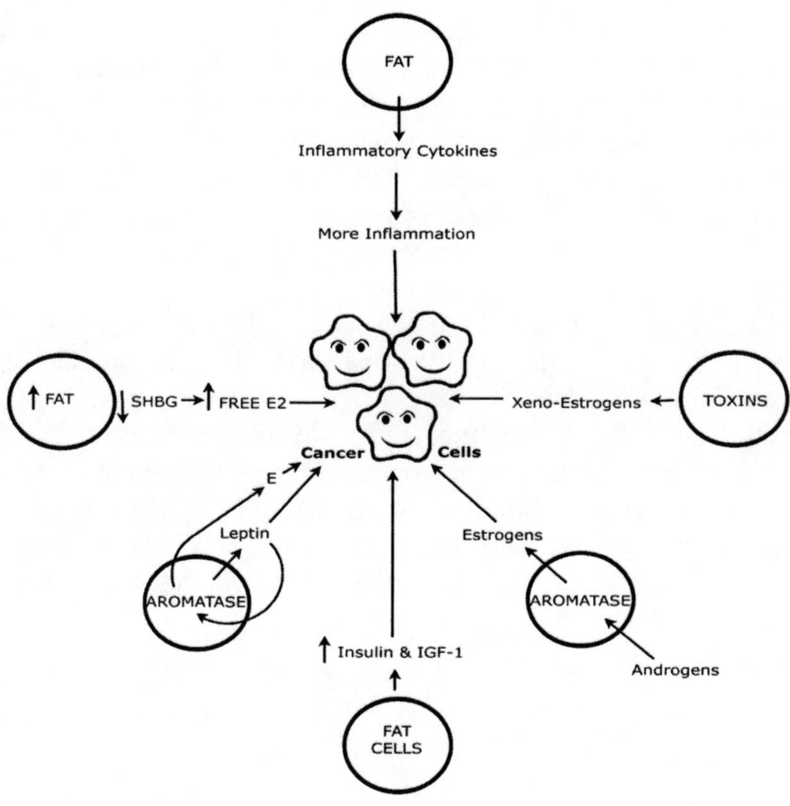

Fig 6—How body fat can stimulate breast cancer growth.

Leptin, another hormone with multiple biological actions, is produced by the adipose (fat) tissue. Its levels rise in people with increased body fat. Leptin has been shown to directly stimulate the growth of cancer cells.[56] Indirectly, it induces the activity of aromatase, thus leading to more estrogen production, a double whammy!

Most of the estrogen in our circulation is bound to a protein, ***Sex Hormone Binding Globulin (SHBG)***. Obesity leads to reduction of SHBG. In other words, the amount of free estrogen is increased. It is free estrogen that is active and stimulates breast cancer cells.[57] Lower SHBG leads to higher free estrogen levels which increase promotion of breast cancer.

Over one hundred studies have looked at the relationship between excess weight and breast cancer.[58] Taken together, they suggest that overweight or obese women have 30% to 50% greater risk of post-menopausal breast cancer than leaner women. Teenage obesity does not have this effect.[59] The reason may be that teenage fat does not produce much estrogen. The effect seems to emerge if excess fat continues beyond the teenage years, which unfortunately happens to most obese teenaged girls.

Excess body fat is a significant cause of many illnesses that affect us in our 40s, 50s and beyond. Women who continuously gain weight throughout life have a high risk of breast cancer. On the other hand, losing weight at any age leads to a reduction in risk of this disease. Losing fat is complex and a difficult process. I spend a great deal of time with my patients on this issue. I have suggested a few ways to reduce body fat and insulin in chapter 6 and will further detail my approach for weight reduction in the final section of this book.

Chapter 9
Alcohol

I am forbidden sugar, fat and alcohol. So hooray, I guess, for oatmeal, lemon juice and chicken soup —Mason Cooley

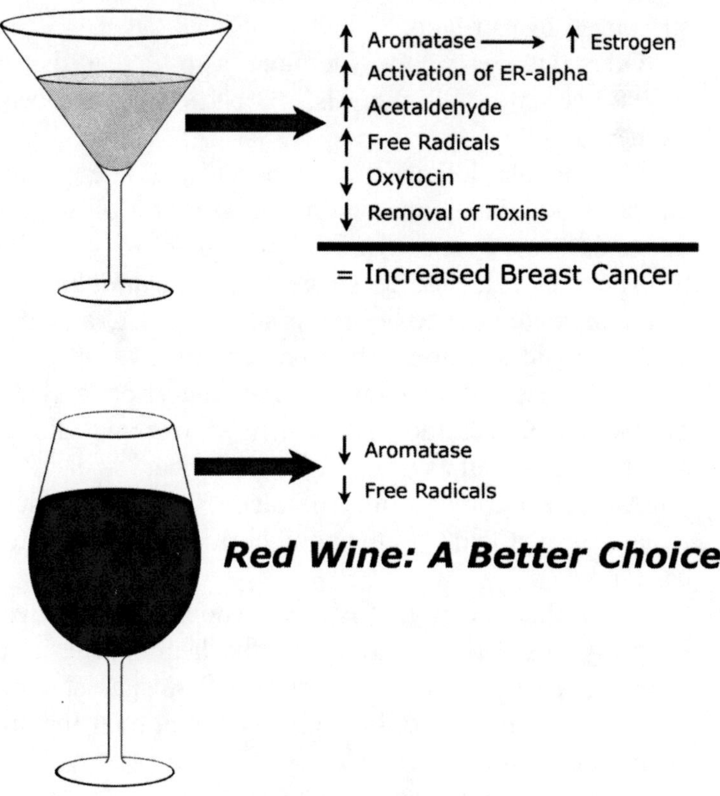

Fig 7—How alcohol can promote breast cancer

Heavy alcohol use has long been known to cause liver disease and increase the risk of cancer of the esophagus, pharynx and liver. Data collected during the last two decades shows that it also increases the risk of breast cancer.[60] One combined analysis of 53 studies from around the world has estimated that one alcoholic drink per day increases the risk of breast cancer by 7%.[61]

Several mechanisms may be in action to explain the stimulatory effect of alcohol on breast cancer (Fig 7).

It has been demonstrated that ethanol can more than double the activity of aromatase in breast cancer cells (MCF-7 cells) grown in dishes in a lab.[62] The same study also showed that alcohol increased estrogen receptor alpha (ER alpha) activity in these cells. Most breast cancers are estrogen receptor positive; they have the estrogen receptor alpha (***ER alpha***) on their surface. Therefore, the more ER alpha activity, the more such cancer cells will be stimulated by estrogen.

Other studies in the literature also reveal that alcohol can increase serum estradiol levels,[63, 64] particularly in post-menopausal women.

Nutritional deficiencies, especially folate deficiency, may enhance the breast cancer stimulating effect of alcohol,[65] perhaps due to decreased capacity of the liver to detoxify carcinogens.

There is evidence to suggest that ***acetaldehyde*** formed as a result of alcohol metabolism binds to DNA, and destructs folic acid. It would therefore act as a carcinogen.

It has been shown that alcohol ingestion may lead to more production of free radicals, which, as we have discussed before, can initiate as well as promote breast cancer.[66]

Another indirect effect of alcohol is that it suppresses the release of oxytocin,[16, 67] the good hormone that can protect us from cancer.

Does this mean that women should totally avoid alcohol? Probably not. One has to weigh the health benefits of moderate drinking, particularly the heart benefits, against the risks. Such benefits have been detailed in a recent National Institute of Health position paper on the topic.[68]

One also has to weigh risk/benefits in light of one's personal lifestyle and social circumstances. I believe that if one wants to drink, it is a good idea to drink red wine in moderate amounts. Red wine has additional benefits. It is a strong anti-oxidant, and, unlike other types of alcohol, actually inhibits aromatase.[69]

- Section 3 -
Inhibition of Breast Cancer

Chapter 10
Estrogens that Inhibit Promotion of Breast Cancer: Estriol and 2-hydroxyestrone

In chapter 4, I described the importance of estrogen for most organ systems of a woman's body, and bemoaned the fact the some estrogens (estrone, estradiol and 16 alpha-hydroxyestrone) can promote the growth of existing breast cancer cells. Now, let us look at the balance that Nature has provided: some estrogens that prevent the promotion of breast cancer. Estriol and 2-hydroxyestrones are two such estrogens.

Estriol (E3) is derived from estradiol (E2) and estrone (E1). It can occupy estrogen receptors on the cancer cells — the sites where estrogen attaches — and thus prevent E2 and E1 from getting in and promoting the growth of these cells.

Normally estriol levels are higher during the leuteal phase (last two weeks of the menstrual cycle) than during the follicular phase (first two weeks). After menopause the levels of estriol tend to drop. Estriol administration to menopausal women improves hot flashes, night sweats and insomnia. It also improves lower urinary-genital symptoms in menopausal women and the health of the vaginal lining. Estriol cream improves elasticity and thickness of the skin and can reduce wrinkles and pore size.

The late Dr. Henry Lemon, former head of the department of Gynecologic Oncology at the University of Nebraska, College of Medicine, spent most of his professional life studying estriol. As far back as the mid 60s, he had shown that women with breast cancer produced less estriol than normal women by measuring the relative amounts of different estrogens in their urine.[70] He also showed that estriol was protective against several chemical carcinogens used to induce breast cancer in laboratory animals.[71, 72] In addition, he found that radiation caused breast cancer in these animals, and that if he gave these animals estriol, he could block the development of breast cancer.

Asian women, who have less breast cancer than American women, generally have higher estriol levels than American women, who instead have higher estradiol and estrone levels. It is also known that fullterm pregnancy provides protection from breast cancer, in spite of the fact that hormone levels are extremely high during pregnancy. The reason is that estriol, progesterone and human chorionic gonadotropins (other protective hormones) are produced in large amounts during pregnancy. Particularly, estriol has been known to increase as much as 1000 fold during this time of a woman's life.

In 2002, Pentii K. Siiteri, PhD, presented hormonal findings on a subset of 15,000 women who were followed for up to 40 years at the California Kaiser Foundation Health Plan. The subset had become pregnant between 1959 and 1967. Their serum samples were saved and stored at—20 degrees C. Of these women, 204 women eventually developed breast cancer. They were compared with 434 who did not. Women with cancer had lower estriol levels during their pregnancies than those who did not. Data analysis revealed that the highest estriol group had 58% less risk of this cancer than the lowest estriol group. These findings were presented at the Department of Defense Breast Cancer Research Meeting in Orlando, FL on September 30, 2002.[73]

There seems to be no question that estriol provides protection against breast cancer. It is unfortunate that traditional HRT has never included estriol. Since the publication of the results of the Women's Health Initiative (WHI) studies, the use of Premarin and all HRT has declined. A few other preparations are being marketed including estradiol patches, which I believe are better than Premarin. Still, the mainstream estrogen therapy continues to exclude estriol.

Whenever I prescribe estrogen for menopausal women, I always include estriol. In fact, my estrogen prescriptions contain 4 times as much estriol as estradiol. I only prescribe natural bio-identical hormones and administer those in natural ways, mimicking the natural release of hormones from the ovaries.

Most physicians prescribing natural bio-identical hormones usually include estriol. Many of them belong to the American

Academy of Anti-Aging Medicine (A4M). You can locate one in your area by logging on to www.worldhealth.net/.

2-hyrdoxyestrone is an important estrogen, a metabolite (product of metabolism) of estradiol. In chapter 4, I explained that estradiol, the most active and important estrogen in humans, changes into two important metabolites: 16 alpha hydroxyestrone and 2-hydroxyestrone. The former promotes the growth of breast cancer cells; the later inhibits it. In other words, 2-hydroxyestrone is a beneficial estrogen. Like estriol, it is a weak estrogen. It blocks the stimulatory action of strong estrogens on ER alpha on breast cancer cells.

Many researchers have found the protective effect of 2-hydroxyestrone and labeled it a 'good'estrogen.[74] According to several studies, a low 2/16 ratio spells higher incidence of post-menopausal breast cancer.[32]

A large Italian study of 10,786 women, the "Hormones and Diet in the Etiology of Breast Cancer" (ORDET) study, has provided conclusive evidence in favor of 2-hydroxyestone. It showed that pre-menopausal women with the highest 2/16 ratio had a 42% reduction in the occurrence of breast cancer compared to those with the lowest 2/16 ratios.[75] These data have been corroborated by others workers.

Generally speaking, healthy diets with low fat (saturated and omega 6) and high vegetables and fruits move the 2/16 E ratio in the right direction. So do certain supplements such as Indole 3 Carbinol, which is also found in cruciferous vegetables. Indole 3 Carbinol has many other anti-breast cancer actions that I will discuss in a later chapter.

Chapter 11
Progesterone

Our remedies oft in ourselves do lie— William Shakespeare

Progesterone is a good hormone. It is brain healthy, heart healthy and bone healthy. More relevant to this topic, it is an anti-cancer hormone.

Progesterone is made from pregnenolone, which in turn is derived from cholesterol. It is mostly synthesized in the ovary, but also in the adrenal gland where it is a precursor to the formation of cortisol. In the ovary it is mostly produced during the second half of the menstrual cycle after ovulation. After an egg is released from a follicle in the ovary, the the follicle turns into a "corpus luteum," which produces progesterone and is the main source of this hormone during the second half of the menstrual cycle. Progesterone prepares the lining of the uterus for implantation of a fertilized egg. It has many actions that tend to counter the effects of estrogen. For example, estrogen stimulates the growth and division of breast and uterine cells. Progesterone opposes these effects and makes these cells look more mature and normal. Estrogen retains fluid in the body; progesterone is a natural diuretic. Estrogen causes anxiety; progesterone creates calmness by its action on the so called GABA receptors in the brain. Estrogen prevents loss of bone; progesterone stimulates new bone formation. Like estrogen it is heart healthy and prevents coronary spasm. It can reduce cravings for sweets, help use fat for energy production, promote sleep and improve libido. It is a very important hormone.

Surgeons and oncologists have known that women who have breast cancer surgery during the first two weeks of their menstrual cycle (follicular phase), tend to have more recurrence, metastases and shorter survival than women who have their surgery during the last two weeks of their cycle (leuteal phase). You would wonder why that is so? The first 14 days are characterized by high circulating un-opposed estrogen, while it is opposed by high levels of progesterone during the last 14 days.[76] Estrogen (estradiol and estrone) would stimulate the growth of any cancer cells dislodged during surgery, whereas progesterone would tend to inhibit it.

I have previously mentioned that women who have had full term pregnancies have less breast cancer. One of the reasons for this protection is the high level of estriol during pregnancy. But, equally important, women have high levels of circulating progesterone during pregnancy, which is inhibitory to breast cancer.

Some years ago, a prospective epidemiological study conducted at Johns Hopkins revealed the importance of progesterone against breast cancer. In this landmark study, 1083 infertile women were followed for 13 to 33 years. They were divided into two groups according to the cause of infertility: endogenous progesterone deficiency or non-hormonal causes. The women in the low progesterone group eventually developed 5 times as much breast cancer as those with normal progesterone. Not only that, the low progesterone group had a 10 fold increase in death rate from all types of cancers when compared to women who had a normal progesterone level.[77]

How does progesterone inhibit growth of breast cancer?

Dr. Ben Formby and T.S. Wiley of Sansum Medical Research Institute, Santa Barbara, CA., have looked into the mechanisms. They studied the effect of progesterone on ***progesterone receptor (PR)*** positive and PR negative tumor cells. They found that progesterone inhibited the proliferation of several lines of human breast cancer cells that were PR positive, but not those which were PR negative. This effect is the reverse of estrogen (estradiol), which stimulates the growth of estrogen receptor positive breast cancer cells. Drs. Formby and Wiley found that progesterone upregulated (enhanced) the ***p53 gene***, a tumor suppressive gene, and down regulated ***bcl-2 and survivin***, the tumor promoting genes. The result was an increased ***'apoptosis' or programmed suicide*** of breast cancer cells.[78, 79] In other words, progesterone helped kill off these cancer cells.

Progesterone is also protective against endometrial (uterus) cancer and perhaps prostate and other cancers. In a study reported from Japan, progesterone even induced apoptosis in mesothelioma, a rare tumor of the lining of the lung.[80]

As opposed to progesterone, **progestins** such as **Provera** (medroxy-progesterone) are artificial molecules that are chemically different from progesterone. They actually increase the risk of breast cancer. This has been demonstrated in large studies in the US and Europe.[27, 28]

Progestins have toxicities that have been well documented over the years. Provera has been shown to cause damage to the lining of blood vessels in young women,[81] which would create a state of inflammation in the vessels. Provera constricts blood vessels rather than dilating those like natural progesterone.[82] It increases atherosclerosis[83] and promotes insulin resistance.[83, 84] Ironically, Provera tends to have an inhibitory effect on the cell division of breast cancer cells in cultures.[85] But it's overall effects in the body, including inflammation and insulin resistance and other, as-yet-undemonstrated effects, increase risk of breast cancer in real life.

A recently reported large French study analyzed the risk of breast cancer among 54,548 post menopausal women on HRT according to the types of hormones used. The data revealed that the relative risk of breast cancer among women receiving estrogen plus synthetic progestin was 1.4 compared to 1 in non-users. In other words, there was a 40% increase in breast cancer. On the other hand among women who used estrogen plus natural progesterone, the relative risk was 0.9 — an actual 10% decrease! There is no question that natural progesterone protected these women from any cancer stimulatory effect of estrogen.[86]

The irony of all this is that physicians in general consider progestins to be the same thing as progesterone. They use these terms interchangeably. Some time ago, a pharmaceutical company, the makers and marketers of Premarin, found out that Premarin, by stimulating the lining of the uterus, was causing uterine cancer in some women. They knew that progesterone could inhibit this effect of Premarin. But progesterone, a natural molecule, cannot be patented. Quite understandably, the drug company altered the molecule to make the patentable medroxy-progesterone (Provera) and called it a progestin. Over time the difference between progesterone and progestin blurred. Even smart doctors consider these substances to be one and the same. I did that too — until I had the good fortune of becoming deeply involved in this subject.

The bottom line is that only natural progesterone has anti-breast cancer effects. Progestin, the artificial progesterone, can actually promote breast cancer.

Progesterone, of any kind, has often been excluded from HRT for women. This is particularly true for women who have had a hysterectomy. These women are surprised to hear that they need progesterone, because they have been told that once the uterus is gone there is no purpose for progesterone — as if the uterus was the only reason nature created progesterone. The fact is that, like all other hormones, progesterone was created for the entire woman.

Chapter 12
Melatonin

In all things of nature there is something of the marvelous – Aristotle

Most people have heard about melatonin as a pill to help fight insomnia or jet lag. In fact, it is an important hormone secreted by the pineal gland, situated in the middle part of our brain, behind and in between the eyes. Its secretion is increased by darkness and, coinciding with deep sleep, peaks around 2 AM. It is inhibited by light, any kind of light, natural or artificial. It is made from tryptophan, which is first converted into serotonin, then into melatonin. Tryptophan is found in many foods, particularly in milk and turkey; hence the need for a nap after a big Thanksgiving dinner.

Melatonin helps set our sleep-wake cycle (circadian rhythm). Talking to other hormones, which rise and fall according to this 24hr cycle, it sets the body's internal biological clock. It is thought to have an effect on the hypothalamus and the pituitary glands (thus affecting most other hormones in the body) and an influence on the thymus gland, the gland that is central to the development and proper functioning of our immune system.

Melatonin secretion starts to decline after age 15. By age 30 we produce less than half, and by age 60 less than one tenth of that from our youth. As melatonin declines, our thymus gland begins to shrink and it all but disappears by age 60. Melatonin has an important role in the modulation of our immune system. As it declines, our immune system also declines and malfunctions with advancing years.

Dr Pierpaoli (Biancalana-Masera Foundation for the Aged, Neuroimmunomodulation Laboratory, Ancona, Italy) and Dr. Lisnikov (Institute of Experimental Medicine, Russian Academy of Medical Science, St.Petersburg) have been pioneers in the study of the pineal gland and melatonin. They demonstrated that transplanting young mice's pineal glands into old mice made the old mice act younger and live longer. On the other hand, transplantation of old pineal glands into younger mice made them appear older and die faster.[87] Drs Pierpaoli's and Lisnikov's 30-year work shows that melatonin plays an extremely important role in the integrity of the neuroendocrine and immune systems.[88, 89]

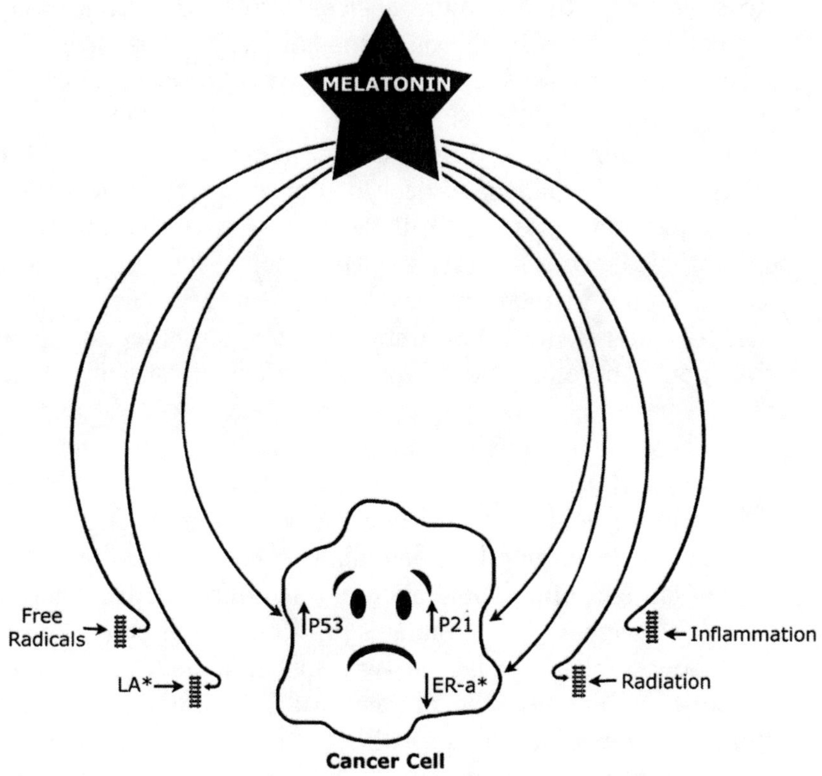

Fig. 8—Inhibitory effects of melatonin on breast cancer

It is logical to conclude that anything that maintains the integrity of our immune system should protect us from cancer. In fact, there is scientific evidence that melatonin protects us against breast cancer, and against cancer in general.

Observational and epidemiological studies show that the incidence of breast cancer is low in blind women, who, because of lack of exposure to light, have higher levels of melatonin. On the contrary, night shift workers such as nurses, flight attendants, radio and telephone operators, have prolonged exposure to light, lower melatonin levels and therefore more breast cancer.[90, 91] Similarly, researchers have shown that melatonin inhibits the growth of experimental breast cancer in rodents, and the growth of human breast cancer cells in culture dishes. Early human cancer studies, combining melatonin with other modalities, such as chemotherapy agents and ***interleukin-2*** (an immune enhancer) have shown encouraging results.[92]

In addition to its immune enhancing effect, several other actions of melatonin have been demonstrated that are anti-breast cancer in nature (see fig 8). It has been shown that melatonin, at physiological concentrations: (a) directly inhibits cancer cell proliferation, (b) increases the tumor suppressor genes, p53 and p21, (c) reduces the concentration of estrogen receptor alpha (ER alpha) and, therefore, the stimulatory effect of estradiol on cancer cells.[93]

Another way in which melatonin helps is by counteracting ***linoleic acid (LA).*** LA, an essential fatty acid, is abundantly present in all vegetable oils, and has tumor promoting properties. In several cancer models, including breast cancer, it has been shown that LA, after being taken into the tumor cells, changes into a growth factor, which stimulates proliferation of cells and growth of cancer. Studies have shown that melatonin is extremely effective in blocking the entrance of LA into tumor cells and, therefore, impeding the growth of cancer cells. In these same studies, constant exposure to light, which reduces natural release of melatonin, markedly increased the uptake of LA into tumor cells and increased tumor growth.[94, 95] It is not surprising why night shift workers have more breast cancer.

Melatonin has been shown to be protective against the effects of radiation.[96] It is well known that radiation is responsible for the occurrence of many cancers. Melatonin helps activate the DNA repair enzymes.

We have discussed before that free radicals are important in the initiation and promotion of breast cancer. Melatonin is a strong natural scavenger of free radicals. It mops them up. Not only that, it increases the production of naturally occurring anti-oxidants inside our cells such as ***super oxide dismutase, glutathione and catalase***.[97] By doing so, it not only prevents cancer, but also many neuro-degenerative diseases such as Alzheimer's disease and Parkinsonism.[98]

We know that inflammation promotes cancer. Melatonin has an anti-inflammatory action.[99]

Melatonin also improves the function of ***mitochondria***, the energy-generating machines in our cells.[100] All life functions depend on the energy fuel produced in our mitochondria. It is called ***ATP***. An average man produces and consumes approximately 100 lbs of ATP per day!! It is an amazing power generating system. But our mitochondria deteriorate as we age. They produce less energy and leak more free radicals with advancing years. This is why melatonin is so important.

I believe that melatonin is not just an anti-cancer agent, it is a natural and overall anti- aging molecule. It is cheap and available in every drug store. It is well tolerated by most people. Rarely, it may cause drowsiness or irritability in a few people. I usually advise a combination of short acting and long acting melatonin, to mimic the natural secretion of melatonin at night.

Chapter 13
DHEA and Testosterone

DHEA

DHEA (dyhydroepiandrosterone) is the most abundant steroid hormone in the body. It is produced by the adrenal gland. In the body we can manufacture other steroid hormones from DHEA, such as testosterone and estrogen. We have high levels of DHEA in our youth, but after age 25 the levels begin to decline. By the time of menopause, women have only one fourth of what they had in their prime.

DHEA has received tremendous attention during the past 20 years. It has been considered to be the 'fountain of youth,' the 'miracle molecule,' the 'grace factor,' and more.

It has been shown to boost our immune response by increasing the number and function of the natural killer cells, prevent heart disease, Alzheimer's, osteoporosis and even cancer.

In 1994, researchers from the University of California, School of Medicine, La Jolla, published a six month study of the effect of DHEA in 30 men and women between the ages of 40 and 70. Each man or woman received DHEA for a while and was crossed over to placebo (fake pill) without their knowledge and without the knowledge of the researchers ***(double blind, cross-over, controlled trial).*** The results showed that while on DHEA 67% of the men and 84% of the women perceived a remarkable increase in their physical and psychological well being. DHEA increased the testosterone levels in women, but had no effect on the estrogen levels.[101] Other studies have shown that DHEA reduces ***visceral*** (abdominal) fat and decreases insulin resistance.[102]

Interestingly, the role of DHEA in breast cancer is complex. I believe it can be a double-edged sword. Too little or too much DHEA can be bad when it comes to breast cancer. Let us look at the evidence.

In 1997, researchers at the CHUL Research Center, Quebec, Canada, reported the protective effects of DHEA against breast cancer in rats. The animals were given DMBA, a poison that caused breast cancer in these rats. One group of rats was then given different doses of DHEA and the other served as a ***control*** (comparison) group. On the average, breast cancer was decreased by 50% in the animals who received DHEA.[103]

Dr. J.E. Green and colleagues from the Laboratory of Cell Regulation and Carcinogenesis, National Cancer Institute, Bethesda, Maryland, reported similar findings in 2001.[104] They studied the effect of DHEA supplementation on breast cancer prone mice, and found that DHEA reduced tumor growth by 50%. They concluded that DHEA had an "inhibitory effect on tumor growth and progression."

Other workers from the National Cancer Institutes (Couillard and associates) showed that even human breast cancer, when transplanted onto mice, was significantly inhibited by DHEA.[105]

In spite of all this favorable scientific evidence, one has to remember that DHEA can change to testosterone, which can further evolve to estrogen. Therefore, one should assume that too much DHEA could, in the end, stimulate breast cancer cells. In fact, it has been demonstrated to do so. If you have human breast cancer cells growing in a culture dish and soak them with large amounts of DHEA, in about 4 days, a significant amount of testosterone and estrogen will form in the dish. The estrogen will then start stimulating the breast cancer cells.[106]

Similar data in humans suggests that low DHEA is related to pre-menopausal breast cancer, where as high serum levels of DHEA are associated with post-menopausal breast cancer.[107]

Dr. Lissoni and colleagues from Milan, Italy, looked at the DHEA levels in 70 cancer patients, including 24 breast cancer patients. They found that patients whose cancer metastasized (spread) had low DHEA levels. Cancer did not seem to spread in those patients whose DHEA levels were normal.[108]

On the other hand, researchers at the National Cancer Institute, Bethesda, Maryland found that women with the highest DHEA level had more breast cancer than those with normal levels. They followed post-menopausal blood donors for up to 10 years to get these results.[109]

Some authorities are quite bullish on the use of DHEA. They argue that at a molecular level, DHEA and its derivative, testosterone, are inhibitory to breast cancer cells. Not only that, they cite the fact that DHEA stimulates bone formation, strengthens vaginal mucosa and decreases insulin resistance, and should therefore be given to post-menopausal women.[110, 111] Others are not too sure. They worry that prolonged use of DHEA may stimulate breast cancer and suggest caution in its use, especially in obese women, who tend to have more aromatase, converting testosterone into estrogen.[112]

So what is the reader to do? If you have too little, you are in trouble, if you have too much, you are in trouble! My answer is to use caution. If your DHEA level is low, bring it up to an average level, by taking as little as necessary.

I routinely check DHEA levels in all menopausal women who come to see me for natural bio-identical hormone replacement therapy. I find it to be low, or towards the lower end of the range, in approximately 70% of such women, and I cautiously correct this deficiency. It improves their sense of well being and energy level. However, I check the levels from time to time and make sure that the levels do not rise above the 60th percentile of the normal range.

Testosterone

DHEA and progesterone can both covert to testosterone. Testosterone is further transformed (by the enzyme aromatase) into estrogen, mostly in the ovaries in pre-menopausal women, and predominantly in fat cells in post-menopausal women. Menopausal women with excessive body fat tend to make more estrogen from testosterone. Some studies suggest that increased levels of testosterone and estrogen are associated with an increased risk of breast cancer.[113] However, if the estrogen level is taken out of the picture, testosterone shows little risk of increasing breast cancer. A recent study on the risk of breast cancer and sex hormones published in the Journal of the National Cancer Institute just proved this.[114] Among 624 women with breast cancer, androgens (testosterone and DHEA), were found not to have added to the risk of breast cancer.

Other investigations have recently revealed that testosterone may actually block the cancer promoting effects of estrogen. A study performed at the National Institute of Health, Maryland, found that estrogen normally induced proliferation of the breast epithelial cells in monkeys. The addition of normal physiologic doses of testosterone almost completely abolished this proliferation. The researchers found that testosterone reduced the estrogen receptor (ER) alpha on these cells, explaining this cancer preventive effect of testosterone.[115] Studies done at the University of Calabria, Italy, also show that testosterone and its final derivative, dihydrotestosterone (DHT) act through an androgen receptor (AR) and inhibit the growth of breast cancer cells in culture dishes.[116]

The question is: should menopausal women receive testosterone? The answer appears to be in the affirmative, if their testosterone level is low or towards the lower end of the laboratory range. Frequently, such women will have low libido, vaginal dryness, a tendency towards osteoporosis and impaired cognition. Testosterone would counteract all of these changes and would be indicated for such women.[117] I have many women in my practice whose muscle tone came back after years of dormancy. Their personal trainers could not believe how their muscles were beginning to "ripple." Some told me that their husbands were surprised how accurately and how long they were hitting the golf ball. Testosterone does not just increase muscle strength and tone, it improves hand-eye coordination.

Again, it is my belief that such supplementation with testosterone should be done cautiously, with natural testosterone, and with follow up checks on testosterone levels. I have seen women who get carried away with the use of testosterone, because it improves libido and sexual function. If the testosterone levels get too high, there will likely be more conversion into estrogen, and that would be undesirable.

Chapter 14
Human Growth Hormone (HGH): "Fountain of Youth"

On July 5,1990, Daniel Rudman, M.D., and his associates from the University of Wisconsin, published an article in the New England Journal of Medicine that ushered in a new era in the history of medicine . . . an entirely new field called "Anti-Aging Medicine" was born. Daniel Rudman gave human growth hormone to men between the ages of 60 and 80 for six months to see if it had any effect on their body fat and musculature. He found that their muscle mass increased by 9%, body fat decreased by 14%, skin thickness increased by 7% and bone density increased by 1.6%. The men felt, acted and looked "10 years younger" and their wives vouched for this regained youth.[118]

This new information convinced some forward-thinking doctors that aging could be slowed or even reversed. They did not want to accept aging in the usual sense. They no longer wanted to tell a 50-year old complaining of diminishing energy: "It's OK for your age, just learn to live with it."

In 1993, 12 such doctors met in Chicago and started the American Academy of Anti-Aging Medicine. Since then, the academy has grown exponentially. As of 2004, there are more than 14,000 doctors and scientists from 70 different countries who are members. The interest in the field and the growth of this specialty of medicine have been phenomenal.

In the beginning, human growth hormone was 'it,' the 'star,' the 'fountain of youth.' All people going through anti-aging were on it. But, as time has passed, things have evolved. We have learned more, and continue to learn more every day.

I believe that aging and age-related diseases are based on different erosive or degenerative mechanisms which affect different people differently. Hormonal imbalance is one of these mechanisms and growth hormone is just one of the several important hormones that decline with age. It is my philosophy to investigate each patient for the known mechanisms of aging, and then create a specific anti-aging program for that person, which may or may not include human growth hormone.

Human growth hormone has many actions or functions. Most of these happen through IGF-1 (insulin like growth factor) which HGH creates as it reaches the liver. Our pituitary gland releases a lot of growth hormone when we are younger, but less and less as we age. We make 500 micrograms per day in our teens, mostly during deep sleep at night. By age 40, we produce 200 micrograms per day, and by age 80, only 25 micrograms.

HGH and IGF-1 deficiency have been associated with a shortened life span[119, 120]; there is no question that HGH is important for health, vigor and vitality. Extensive scientific research continues to demonstrate the many benefits of HGH, which include:

- Better mood
- Clarity of mind
- Improved musculature
- Decreased body fat
- Increased bone density
- Better skin
- Better immune system
- Re-growth of vital organs
- Better wound healing
- More energy and sense of well being and drive

Despite all of these benefits there is a fear, among physicians and lay people alike, that HGH may cause cancer. The fear is exaggerated, unjustified and without scientific basis. Let us look at the evidence.

IGF-1, the important derivative of HGH, is a growth factor. It makes cells grow, including cancer cells.[121] It has been shown in cell culture dishes that IGF-1 stimulates the proliferation of breast cancer cells acting in conjunction with estradiol.[122] A multiple center study led by Dr. Susan Hankinson from Brigham and Women's Hospital and Harvard Medical School, which included 397 women with breast cancer, revealed that high IGF-1 levels were associated with increased breast cancer in pre-menopausal women, but not in post menopausal women.[123] But most such studies reveal that a protein that naturally binds IGF-1 in the blood, called ***IGFBP-3*** (insulin-like growth factor binding protein-3) is also low in such patients. This scenario is especially common in people with insulin resistance.

IGFBP-3 is a protective protein with anti-cancer activities. It has been shown to inhibit the estrogen induced proliferation of breast cancer cells.[124] It also causes what is called programmed death (apoptosis) of breast cancer cells.

What is important to know is the fact that when human growth hormone is given to patients, it does not just increase IGF-1; it also increases IGFBP-3, so that the cancer stimulating and cancer inhibiting effects tend to cancel each other. In addition, there are other ***anti-cancer effects of growth hormone*** that have been revealed by scientific research (fig 9):

1. It has been demonstrated that growth hormone repairs DNA damage caused by radiation and other toxic agents.[125] As we have discussed before, DNA damage is at the root of all cancers.
2. HGH increases the activity of Natural Killer cells.[126] Natural Killer cells are our first defense against cancer. They constantly patrol the body looking for any foreign material, such as virus or cancer cells. Upon finding such cells they immediately inject powerful enzymes to destroy the 'enemy.'
3. HGH promotes the proliferation of the cells of our thymus gland (which naturally shrinks as we age). It modulates the secretion of thymic hormones and over-all immune function, a necessary defense against cancer.[127]
4. It improves multiple other aspects of our immune function,[128] including the function of cells called monocytes, further fortifying our defenses against cancer.[129]
5. Growth hormone increases the production of ***glutathione***, a cellular anti-oxidant, which inhibits "***Nuclear Factor Kappa B***," a factor that controls the cell's survival genes. When that happens, cancer cells undergo programmed cell death (apoptosis) or suicide.[130]
6. Growth hormone administration leads to increased levels of vitamin D in the blood.[131] As we will discuss later, vitamin

D has important anti-cancer actions.

7. Low dose growth hormone reduces visceral fat and insulin resistance.[132] As we already know, visceral fat and insulin resistance both promote breast cancer. So both of these actions should reduce the growth of breast cancer.

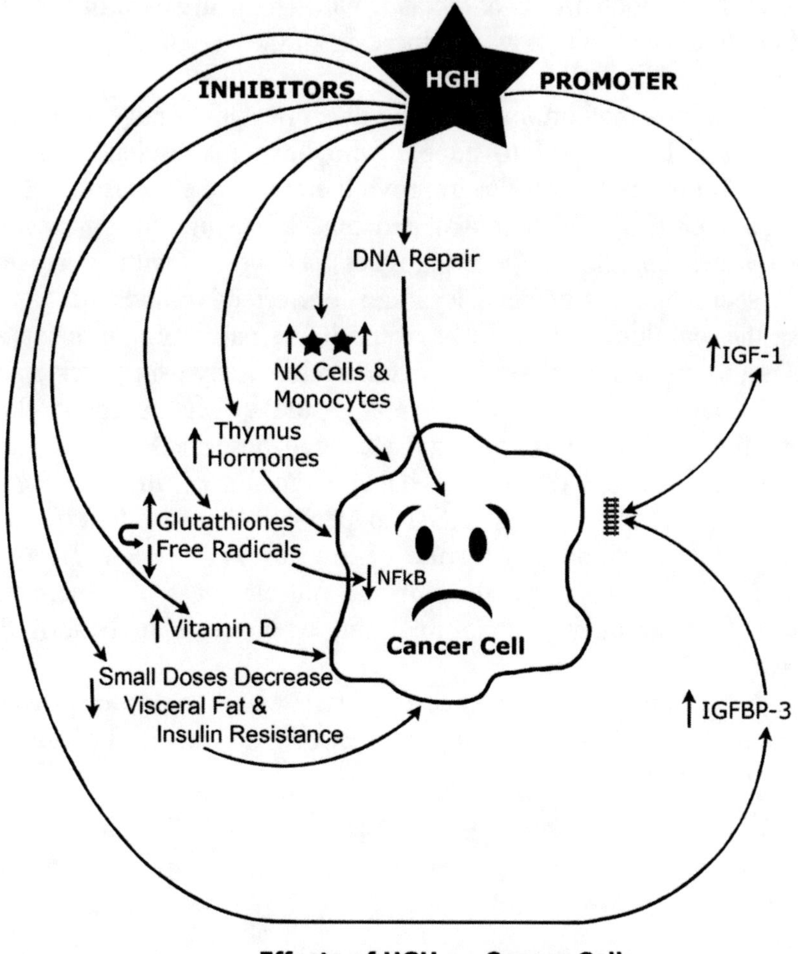

Fig 9—Effects of HGH on Breast Cancer

In other words, the fear of cancer with HGH is just fear. Based on the above evidence, it should not increase cancer, and may even be protective against it.

No studies to date show that growth hormone administration, in adults, poses any risk of breast cancer. In 2003, a western anti-aging clinic presented data at the annual meeting of A4M. Among some 2000 patients who had received HGH over several years, there had been only one case of cancer.

Acromegally, a disease characterized by high secretion of HGH throughout life, is associated with slight increase in the rate of colon cancer, but shows no increase in the rate of cancers of the breast or prostate.[133]

So what's the bottom line? I believe one should not be afraid to give growth hormone to people who have insufficiency of this important hormone. I try to improve the night time release of HGH in such patients, in their 40s and 50s, by using substances that increase such release (secretagogues). However, with increasing age secretagogues become less and less effective and one has to use the real thing, HGH. I like to use it in small morning doses, so as not to disturb its night time natural release. By using such small doses daily, I have never seen any side effects, such as fluid retention or joint pain, which have been described with the un-physiologic large doses of HGH given three times a week. Generally, I avoid giving HGH to people who are already lean, muscular and vigorous, in spite of low levels of IGF-1. It is the patient who is tired, has diminished muscle mass and increased body fat, particularly abdominal fat, who seems to benefit the most.

Again, there is no evidence that HGH causes breast or prostate cancer. It has numerous anti-aging effects and health benefits. It may even prevent cancer.

Chapter 15
Tri-iodothyronine (T3): the Anti-breast Cancer Thyroid Hormone

The thyroid gland makes several hormones. T3 and T4 are the important thyroid hormones, T3 being 5 times as active as T4. These hormones are important for all metabolic functions, reproduction, growth, differentiation and repair of cellular DNA damage. Lower levels of these hormones are associated with fatigue, cold intolerance, weight gain, dry skin, coarse hair, high cholesterol, increased severity of coronary artery disease, mental clarity and even higher mortality among hospitalized patients. The release of these hormones from the thyroid gland is indirectly under the control of the ***hypothalamus*** (hormone control center in the brain) and the ***pituitary*** glands (see fig 10). To simplify things, it works this way. When the body senses deficiency of thyroid hormones (T3 and T4) it sends a signal via the hypothalamus to the pituitary gland to release ***TSH*** (thyroid stimulating hormone), which in turn orders the thyroid gland to make more T3 and T4. On the other hand, when there is too much thyroid hormone in the body, the same signaling process puts the brakes on the release of TSH, so T3 and T4 are adjusted back to normal. This "***negative feedback system***" is important in the physiologic control of thyroid. Most physicians, while checking thyroid, check TSH and maybe T4, but usually ignore T3. It is important to check T3 levels, because there are patients whose TSH and T4 may be normal, but who have low T3. I am emphasizing this because T3 is an important hormone in the defense against breast cancer.

Breast cancer has been found to be associated with several thyroid abnormalities, but most commonly with ***hypothyroidism*** (low thyroid), especially in women who also have an enlargement of thyroid.[134] Studies have shown a significant relationship of breast cancer with low T3, but not with T4 or TSH.[135] This relationship is generally not appreciated by the medical community. However, the medical literature contains many studies that reveal the protective actions of T3 against breast cancer:

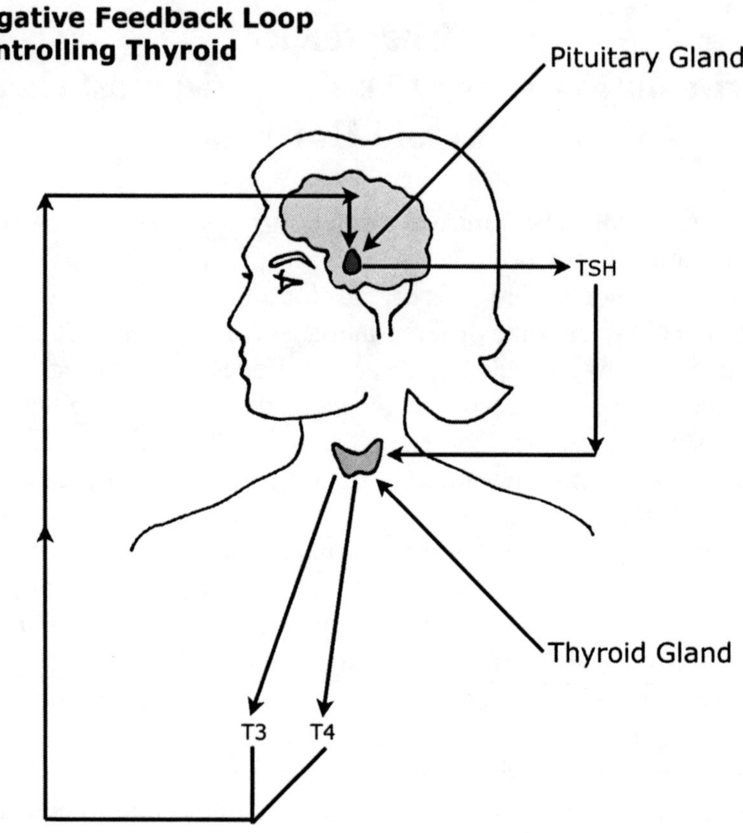

Fig 10—Negative Feedback Loop Controlling Thyroid Hormone Release

1. It is known that as we age, the activity of our ***Natural Killer (NK)*** cells declines. NK cells are our primary defense against cancer. A study published in the journal Gerontology showed that T3 increases NK activity.[136]
2. A study published in the Endocrinology Journal demonstrated that T3 modulates our immune response. It increased the Interleukin-2 receptor on mono-nuclear cells in the blood.[137] ***Interleukin-2***, a cytokine or humor made by the immune system, is important in our defense against cancer and has been used in several cancer treatment protocols.
3. ***Tenacin-C*** is a protein in the breast cancer cells that stimulates the growth of these cells. A study in Madrid,

Spain, found that T3 down regulated (inhibited) tenacin-C in human breast cancer cells in cultures.[138]

4. ***Cyclin D1 and T1*** are genes that are turned on in several kinds of breast cancer cells. They lead to proliferation of these cells. T3 was found to inhibit these genes.[139]
5. ***MCF-7*** are common breast cancer cells grown in culture dishes. Adding T3 suppresses the growth of these cells.[140]
6. T 3 decreases aromatase activity in cells.[141] As we know, higher aromatase activity increases estrogen production which can stimulate growth of breast cancer cells.
7. Another way T3 can decrease the availability of estrogen to cancer cells is by increasing ***sex hormone binding globulin (SHBG),*** which binds up estrogen. It has been shown to do so in obese women.[142]
8. As we have discussed before, and will discuss further in a subsequent chapter, ***oxytocin*** hormone is protective against breast cancer. T3 has been shown to up regulate (augment) oxytocin gene by five-fold.[143]
9. Both T3 and T4 seem to help ***repair DNA*** as it comes under attack by free radicals.[144]

I have several women patients whose thyroid function had been found to be "normal." However, on checking free T3, I found it to be borderline low to low normal. They had problems like weight gain, high cholesterol, low energy, dry skin and impaired memory. I gave them low doses of Armour thyroid (not Synthroid, which contains only T 4) and brought their T3 levels to the mid range of normal. Almost all of them improved. They became more alert and energetic, their skin and hair improved, their thinking became clearer, even cholesterol declined a bit. It is also very likely that T3 is decreasing their risk of breast cancer.

Chapter 16
Oxytocin: The More-than-lactation Hormone!

No one talks about oxytocin. In medical school you learn about it in your physiology class, just once, as a hormone secreted by the pituitary gland that lets the milk down so a mother can breast feed the baby. Then it is forgotten, forever.

In my 30 plus years of medical practice, attending hundreds of clinical meetings and conferences and reading thousands of articles, I never saw anything on oxytocin until I stumbled upon the writings of Dr. T.G. Murrell, a former member of the Department of Community Medicine, Adelaide University of Australia.[4, 15] Dr. Murell preached that women should have regular stimulation of the breast and nipple to prevent breast cancer.

No one seems to have followed up on his idea. It is such a low-tech and unsophisticated approach that it would not have caught the fancy of our academic researchers, who frequently engage in drug company-sponsored research. There are no shots, no pills, no sales, and no money to be made in a project like this.

Nevertheless, this simple idea makes sense. Let us look at why.

We know that women who breast feed have less breast cancer. The more they breast feed, the less chance of this disease. Studies from 30 different countries have proven this fact.[5] The reason for this protection seems to be the hormone, oxytocin, which is released from the pituitary gland with the cry of a baby and during suckling. It causes contractions in the milk ducts to propel the milk. In other words, it cleans these ducts.

When there has been no lactation for long periods of time, secretions tend to accumulate and stagnate in the milk ducts. As these secretions break down, they release free radicals[3, 4] right next to the cells that line the ducts, cells that most commonly become cancerous in a woman's breast. Free radicals initiate and promote cancer — this is an established fact.

Oxytocin fights breast cancer in additional ways. Acting through its receptor on tumor cells (***OR***), it directly inhibits the growth of breast cancer. Oxytocin also down regulates (inhibits) the ***estrogen receptor alpha*** (ER alpha), which is needed for estrogen to bind and then cause growth of cancer cells.[145]

Other studies indicate that oxytocin may be a universal anti-cancer molecule. Dr. Cassoni and associates from the Department of Biomedical Sciences and Human Oncology, University of Turin, Italy, have found and reported that many types of cancer cells have oxytocin receptors, through which oxytocin exerts its anti-proliferative effect. They found that oxytocin inhibited the growth of cancer cells of the breast, uterus, brain and bone.[146]

Other hormonal research shows that oxytocin decreases the release of ***ACTH*** (***adrenocorticotrophic hormone***) from the pituitary gland. ACTH stimulates the adrenal gland to produce more ***cortisone (the stress hormone***). As the oxytocin level rises the cortisone level falls.[147] In fact, it has been proven that breast feeding reduces stress and negative moods in lactating women.[148] Negative moods inhibit our immune response and may be associated with increased risk of breast cancer. I will come to this point later.

So what does oxytocin have to do with Dr. Murrell's recommendation regarding breast and nipple stimulation? Actually, it has been demonstrated that such stimulation for 10 minutes increases a woman's oxytocin level by up to 100%. It is more effective during the last 2 wks of the menstrual cycle, and is diminished by alcohol.[16]

I encourage my female patients to engage in breast and nipple stimulation on a frequent basis and in a hygienic manner. It is quite likely that this simple technique would reduce the initiation as well as growth of breast cancer.

Chapter 17
SHBG (Sex Hormone Binding Globulin)

SHBG is a protein produced by the liver. It binds the sex hormones such as estrogen and testosterone and carries them in the bloodstream. Most physicians consider it to be just a carrier protein. But, it is more than that. It is a part of the system of checks and balances that nature creates in our bodies to maintain function and optimal health. SHBG prevents breast cancer.

We have known for ages that girls who have an early menarche (start having periods at an early age) have more breast cancer later in life. Most people believe that it is due to the prolonged exposure to high cycling levels of estrogen over many years. But what is commonly not appreciated is that girls with early menarche also have low concentrations of SHBG for years after menarche,[149] thus increasing their risk of cancer.

Dr. Moore JW, and associates, of the Imperial Cancer Research Fund, London, measured SHBG in 5,000 women over the age of 35. They found that women who had late menarche had higher SHBG,[150] which explains why such women have less breast cancer. Dr. Moore also found that SHBG level decreased as body weight increased. It is a well known fact that obese women have low SHBG and higher risk of breast cancer. The same group of researchers also found that breast cancer growth was faster in women with low SHBG than in those with normal levels of this protein.[151]

Another group of investigators from the University of Torino, Italy, found that 25% of patients with estrogen receptor positive breast cancers have ***mutated*** (abnormal) SHBG.[152] These same investigators demonstrated that breast cancer cells have a receptor for SHBG though which SHBG inhibits their proliferation and growth. SHBG also blocks estradiol from fueling these cancer cells.[153]

Insulin decreases the secretion of SHBG. Women with high insulin levels and insulin resistance have low SHBG (and more breast cancer). A French group has characterized low SHBG as a marker of insulin resistance, diabetes and overall mortality in post menopausal women.[154]

To make it short, SHBG is important in the prevention of breast cancer, albeit not very well recognized.

Is there a way to increase SHBG in women? The answer is yes. Regular exercise can help increase SHBG. Also, T3 (the most active thyroid hormone), which fights breast cancer in so many ways, increases SHBG. Research has revealed that giving small doses of T3 to obese women, without a diagnosis of hypothyroidism, increases their SHBG levels significantly.[155]

I think overweight women with “low-normal” free T3 levels should receive small doses of Armour thyroid (not synthroid, which contains only T4) to raise their T3 levels to around the middle of the normal range. It will help them improve their metabolism, lose some weight, improve energy for exercise, lower cholesterol, improve their hair and skin, increase their SHBG, and lower the chance of breast cancer.

Chapter 18
Exercise . . . Still the Best Medicine!

All thinking people, even those who don't exercise, know that exercise is good for health. Numerous studies and articles in all languages, all over the world, have attested to these benefits during the last 30 years. A recent update on all scientific studies published between 2000 and 2003 confirms that physical exercise reduces cardiovascular disease, stroke, obesity, diabetes, falls and injuries, mental stress and cancer.[156]

Dr. Lee, of the Department of Preventive Medicine, Brigham and Women's Hospital and Harvard Medical School, recently published a review of all epidemiological studies looking at the role of physical exercise in the prevention of cancer. The results show that there is an overall 30-40% reduction in colon cancer and 20-30% decrease in cancer of the breast.[157]

In 1997, researchers from the University of Tromso, Norway, reported their findings on the role of exercise in breast cancer prevention. They enrolled 25,624 women, aged 20 to 54, in a survey and followed them for 13 years. After adjusting for age and body mass index (weight), they found that exercise reduced the risk of breast cancer by 37%.[158] Women who were lean had added protection.

In 2001, the same researchers compiled the results of 41 studies of 108,031 breast cancer patients, relating risk to physical activity. They concluded that it needs moderate activity (more than 4.5 Metabolic Equivalents or METs) over many years to have significant reduction in risk of breast cancer.[159] Most aerobic workout machines show the METs readings as you work out. Activities that generate more than 4.5 METs include:

- golfing with a pull cart or carrying the bag
- tennis
- jogging
- biking
- aerobic machine workout
- Very brisk walking

A 2004 study from Sweden looked at the effect of exercise during adolescence and early adulthood on risk of subsequent breast cancer. They analyzed 23 such studies and reported that such activity reduced risk of breast cancer by 20%.[160] In other words, any exercise at any period of life is helpful.

How does exercise diminish risk of breast cancer? There seem to be multiple mechanisms involved.

Exercise decreases insulin resistance and decreases insulin level.[161, 162] As I have explained previously, insulin is a growth factor which promotes the proliferation of breast cancer cells. Insulin resistance and high insulin also lead to an inflammatory state in the body, which again promotes breast cancer. Lowering insulin and decreasing insulin resistance is therefore a potent weapon against breast cancer.

Post menopausal women make their estrogen mostly in the fat cells of the body, such as those in the breast. The blood level of estrogen in these women is a reflection of what is being made in the fatty tissue. Breast tissue concentration of estrogen may be 10 to 50 times higher than that in the blood. In post menopausal women, higher blood levels of estrogen are associated with higher risk of breast cancer, thus suggesting that breast levels are proportionally even higher and promoting the growth of adjacent cancer cells. It has been shown that exercise reduces the estrogen levels in post menopausal women,[163] suggesting lower production in the fatty tissue.

Exercise increases sex hormone binding globulin (SHBG), which also fights breast cancer.[164, 165]

Of great interest is the fact that exercise increases the release and levels of growth hormone in men and women,[166, 167] while at the same time lowering IGF-1 (insulin like growth factor-1) levels in those who are losing weight.[168, 169] As I have explained before, growth hormone has many anti-breast cancer effects, while IGF-1 stimulates breast cancer cells. These are exactly the changes one wants to see. Exercise accomplishes both of these.

There is no question, exercise is the best medicine! The problem is that most people can not get around to developing an exercise program for various reasons, be it lack of time, lack of money to join a club or buy home exercise equipment, or just plain lack of energy to exercise. As a rule, I try to uncover the reasons why a particular patient is not exercising. Then I patiently work to remove the obstacles one by one. Many a times, it works; but, frequently there are hurdles. I will summarize my approach in the guidelines at the end of the book.

Chapter 19
All Fats Are Not Created Equal

In chapter 6, we discussed the role of dietary fat in the causation of breast cancer. The main discussion related to inflammation. Saturated fats (animal fats, eggs) and omega 6 polyunsaturated fats (most vegetable oils) can create an inflammatory state in the body. They do this by increasing arachidonic acid (see chapter 6), which produces inflammatory prostaglandin, PG-2. This prostaglandin stimulates aromatase, leading to increased production of estrogen in the tissues. This promotes growth of breast cancer cells.

There are additional mechanisms by which fats promote growth of cancer cells. For example, some studies show that eating beef and pork increases damage to DNA in women, and thereby the risk for cancer; whereas vegetable intake reduces such damage.[170]

Other studies have shown that low fat diets actually reduce estrogen levels in pre-menopausal women,[171] which should reduce their risk. Experimental studies in mice and rats consistently show an increased occurrence of breast cancer with high fat intake.[172]

All of this evidence correlates with the fact that breast cancer is more common in western countries with their high intake of saturated, omega 6 fats and trans-fats, than in countries with low intake of such fats. Still, case-controlled studies in western countries do not support a strong correlation with fat intake.[173] This discrepancy is most likely due to the fact that all fats are not created equal. Some fats are cancer promoting, while others may actually be protective!

Dairy fat is saturated fat. However, it does not seem to increase the risk of breast cancer.[174] The reason seems to be that dairy, in addition to saturated fat, contains vitamin D, which has important anti-cancer effects.

Omega 9 fats, like olive oil, are protective against breast cancer. Researchers, who have looked at the dietary patterns of fat intake in different countries, attest to this fact.[175, 176] Dr. A. Trichopoulou, from the Department of Hygiene and Epidemiology,

University of Athens Medical School, has estimated that liberal olive oil intake can reduce breast cancer by 15%.[177]

DMBA is a poison that has been shown to cause breast cancer in rats. A DMBA study showed that corn oil (omega 6) stimulates growth of such cancer, while olive oil (omega 9) inhibits it.[178]

Omega 3 fats, such as fish oil and flax seed oil, also seem to provide protection against breast cancer. In experimental studies using cultures of breast cancer cells in dishes and human breast cancers transplanted in mice, omega 3 fats inhibit the growth of cancer cells.[179] These same fatty acids can also appear to make breast cancer cells commit suicide (apoptosis).[180]

Unfortunately, case control studies on 'low fat diets' in the prevention of breast cancer have not provided conclusive results. The reasons for such findings are:

a) Some fats promote breast cancer and others protect against it,
b) When you reduce fat, you have to increase something else. If that something happens to be complex carbohydrates with fiber (whole grains and vegetables) and protein, you will reduce breast cancer. If it is simple or refined carbohydrates (sugar, pasta, white bread, white rice), the risk will increase.

Based on up- to-date research, it is my belief that the following statements hold true with regard to dietary fats and risk of breast cancer:

1. Animal fat, from beef and pork, stimulates breast cancer
2. Omega 6 fats (most vegetable oils) stimulate breast cancer if ingested with carbohydrates (inflammatory action) and may inhibit it if taken in with proteins (anti-inflammatory action). If these oils are oxidized (rancid), which they become after prolonged heating or exposure to sun, they generate free radicals which promote cancer
3. Dairy fat has no effect on breast cancer
4. Omega 9 fats (especially olive oil) inhibit breast cancer
5. Omega 3 fats (fish, fish oils, flax seed oil) inhibit breast cancer

To summarize, fats can be good or bad. One should limit

beef and pork fat intake and even the use of vegetable oils. Vegetable oils should be purchased in small bottles, not to last for more than a month, and stored in a cool dark place to avoid oxidation. Prolonged heating, such as deep frying, almost always leads to oxidation. Oxidized oils increase free radicals that lead to aging and all age related diseases including cancer. Vegetable oils become inflammatory when combined with carbohydrates and anti-inflammatory when mixed with proteins. That is why it is important to eat some protein at every meal. Dairy fats are not bad. Butter does not get oxidized during cooking and can be used in moderation. Olive oil should be routinely used in cooking and in salads. Omega 3 fats from cold water deep sea fish, like wild salmon, should be a part of everyone's diet. However, fish has become polluted with mercury, dioxins and PCBs. Therefore, adding good quality fish oil capsules as supplements, to create balance, makes a lot of sense.

Chapter 20
Fruits, Vegetables, Complex Carbohydrates and Soy

A study published in JAMA (Journal of the American Medical Association) looked at the collective results of 8 studies including 351,825 women, 7,377 of whom had breast cancer. They correlated the dietary habits of these women and found that fruit and vegetable intake had no significant effect on the risk of breast cancer.[181]

A blanket statement like this may sway women away from eating fruits and vegetables. It is too simplistic a conclusion and an unfortunate decision. A more logical approach would be to look at all the available evidence.

In reality, the anti-cancer effect depends upon the mix of things that you are eating. If you habitually eat fruits with high ***glycemic index*** (those that raise blood sugar too high), such as ripe bananas and pineapple, you may be raising your insulin levels too much. High insulin, as we have seen before, is a growth factor for breast cancer cells. If, on the other hand, 'fruits and vegetables' means mostly vegetables, you are increasing the intake of fiber, which lowers insulin levels.[182] Similarly, low glycemic fruits like berries, pears, peaches and apples may be quite beneficial because of their anti-oxidant activity and fiber content.

You can get high amounts of fiber from vegetables, certain fruits, and, importantly, from complex carbohydrates. High fiber intake not only lowers insulin, but it also has been shown to lower serum estrogen levels, a definite benefit in breast cancer prevention.[183]

Cruciferous vegetables (broccoli, Brussels sprouts, cabbage, cauliflower) influence the metabolism of estrogen into more favorable estrogen: 2-hydroxyestrone, which is protective against breast cancer. Several studies have shown this to be a fact.[184] Soy has a similar effect on the metabolism of estrogen, changing it into good estrogens.[185] Also, soy ingredients act as weak estrogens and can block estrogen receptors on the cancer cells, thus keeping estradiol and estrone, the stronger stimulating estrogens, away from the cancer cells. Soy consumption is one of the reasons why breast cancer is less common in Japan.

Another reason why the JAMA study did not reveal a benefit from fruits and vegetables has to do with the fact that most supermarket fruits and vegetables consumed in western countries are loaded with pesticides, which, as I have mentioned before, are carcinogenic. Every effort should be made to consume ***organic*** fruits and vegetables.

To summarize, we should use judgment and be appropriately selective. Vegetables are generally all good, but cruciferous varieties are the best. High glycemic fruits should be minimized, and low glycemic fruits encouraged. Every effort should be made to consume only organically grown fruits and vegetables to avoid pesticide. As for carbohydrates, the main focus should be on complex kinds with lots of fiber. Low fiber and refined carbohydrates are glycemic and would cause the same problem as the glycemic fruits, that is, they would raise insulin levels. High insulin is not only implicated in cancer, but in most chronic diseases of aging. I call it the "***Aging Hormone.***"

Chapter 21
Vitamins and Minerals—The Copilots of All Metabolic Functions

Your mother was right when she said, "take your vitamins." Vitamins and minerals are essential for numerous life functions within our cells. Some we can make ourselves, but many of them must enter our bodies through food. However, our modern refining, storing and cooking techniques can strip our food of many of these vital ingredients. This necessitates that we take a vitamin supplement with our food.

Epidemiological studies of vitamins and minerals generally suggest that they provide protection from breast cancer. But some case control studies have yielded conflicting results.

Le Vecchia and associates from Milan, Italy, systematically reviewed data from multiple case control studies conducted in Italy from 1983 to 1999. The data showed that there was significant protection against breast cancer with the use of anti-oxidants, vitamin C, and E and beta carotene. They published their findings in the European Journal of Nutrition in 2001.[186]

Researchers from Johns Hopkins University, Department of Epidemiology, looked at the effect of serum concentrations of vitamin E, beta-carotene and vitamin A among women who donated blood in Washington County in Maryland. After several years, 295 of these women developed breast cancer. They turned out to have significantly lower baseline levels of beta carotene, lycopene, and total carotene, compared with 295 women who did not develop cancer.[187]

Dr. J.F. Dorgan and associates from the National Cancer Institute, Bethesda, Maryland, similarly followed blood donating women for nine and a half years. They found that women with higher levels of certain types of carotenoids, such as ***lycopene*** (found in cooked tomatoes and tomato sauce), had lower occurrence of breast cancer. But they did not find any relationship with beta-carotene (found in carrots), alpha-tocopherol, the usually used form of vitamin E, vitamin A or selenium.[188]

Dr. S.M. Zhang from the division of preventive medicine,

Brigham and Women's Hospital and Harvard Medical School, reviewed English language articles published since August 2002 and reported the findings in Feb of 2004.[189] These studies did not support a protective effect for vitamin C and E, but showed distinct benefit from folate (especially among alcohol users) and vitamin D.

So how do we make sense of all of this information? Let us look at these vitamins separately in light of the scientific evidence.

The role of **vitamin E** has been confusing and complex. The epidemiological studies suggest that dietary vitamin E provides protection against breast cancer, while vitamin E supplements do not.[190] The reason for this discrepancy is that the commonly used vitamin E supplement, ***alpha tocopherol,*** is an incomplete vitamin E. In nature, there are eight vitamin E's, four ***tocopherols*** and four ***tocotrienols,*** all of which are important. However, the medical community has only used alpha tocopherol as a supplement. Early research between 1922 and 1950 showed that alpha tocopherol was the most predominant tocopherol in the body; it was an anti-oxidant and it allowed fertility in laboratory animals. The researchers discounted the rest of the vitamin Es as "minor" and unimportant. From then on all vitamin E supplementation consisted of alpha tocopherol. For many years, physicians like myself, recommended up to 400 international units per day, for health promotion.

In 1997, while attending the annual meeting of the American Academy of Anti-Aging Medicine in Las Vegas, I stopped at a booth where a nutritionist was extolling the virtues of tocotrienols, the minor vitamin E's, most of which were unfamiliar to us. I listened with interest, purchased a bottle and took these vitamin Es for a few months. Then I stopped, not really knowing the scientific basis for what I was doing. But the thought remained with me, that the vitamin E we are using and recommending is incomplete. As time passed, more and more information became available and convinced me that the current vitamin E supplementation was incomplete and un-natural. I switched to the natural (complete) preparation in 2002. By the end of 2004, the American Heart Association was warning against the use of conventional vitamin E (alpha-tocopherol).

Nature does nothing uselessly — Aristotle

In nature, ***gamma tocopherol*** is the major vitamin E in our food. Many studies have revealed that it has some extremely important actions in the body.[191, 192] In particular, it has anti-inflammatory properties and has been shown to improve cardiac health and prevent cancer. Yet, it was never included in vitamin E supplements. What is of real concern is the finding that large doses of alpha tocopherol, the usual vitamin E supplement, deplete the body of gamma tocopherol. That explains why study after study has found "vitamin E" to be of little use in so many aspect of health, including breast cancer prevention.

There is no question in my mind that we need to take complete vitamin E with all its natural components. It is present in nuts and seeds and in newer E preparations containing all the natural ingredients. It never pays to fool with Mother Nature!

Folic acid, or what is commonly referred to as folate, is an important vitamin involved in the synthesis (formation) of DNA. It also repairs the DNA as it comes under attack by free radicals hundreds of times each day.

Some 30 years ago it was believed that the main function of folate was to prevent a kind of anemia called "macrocytic anemia." A few years later it gained reputation for preventing 'neural tube' (nervous system) defects during pregnancy and in the prevention of cardiovascular disease.[193] Then, studies in patients with ulcerative colitis suggested that folate reduced the chance of colon cancer, which is common in patients with this disease.

Finally, epidemiological data has emerged showing that folate is protective against breast cancer. Dr. S. Zhang and associates, at Harvard School of Public Health, conducted an analysis of 88,818 women enrolled in the 1980 "Nurses Health Study." They found that folate reduced the risk of breast cancer among women who consumed one or more alcoholic drinks per day (15 or more grams per day). The risk was reduced by 45% if women took at least 600 micrograms of folate, compared to those who took half or less of that amount.[194] This and other similar studies have been the subject of further reviews, confirming this very important effect of folate against breast cancer.[195] Women who consume alcohol should definitely be taking folate supplements.

Similar to folate is **vitamin B12.** It also has important actions at the DNA level and is known to prevent a kind of macrocytic anemia. In addition, it helps maintain the integrity of our nervous system.

A study from the Vitamin Bioavailability Laboratory, Tufts University, has revealed that in post menopausal women, the risk of breast cancer rises as vitamin B12 level falls,[196] suggesting another important role for B12.

Unfortunately, un-recognized borderline deficiency of B12 is common in aging populations. As we age, the production of acid in our stomachs declines. Since acid is required to split vitamin B12 from food before it can be absorbed into the bloodstream, the blood and tissue levels of B12 also decline. I believe it is good idea for post menopausal women to include vitamin B12 in their daily supplementation.

Vitamin D is an extremely important molecule for all organisms. Animals and plants have been making it upon exposure to the ultra-violet rays of the sun for more than 500 million years. Human beings make 75 to 80 % of our vitamin D this way. The rest comes from food. Food, in fact, is a poor source of vitamin D. Fatty fish has a fair amount. Milk has some, about 100 IU's (international units) per glass. On the other hand, upon total body exposure to sun, we can make as much as 10,000 IU's/day, which confirms that sun exposure is the main source of vitamin D, and that the physiologic limit is 10,000 units per day. The 200 IU contained in the daily quota of over-the-counter calcium pills is simply not enough.[197]

Vitamin D receptors are present in a wide variety of tissues including brain, bone, heart, stomach, intestine, skin, gonads, ***T and B cells*** of our immune system and even many types of cancer cells. According to Dr. Michael Holick, head of the Vitamin D Laboratory, Department of Medicine, Boston University Medical Center, Vitamin D deficiency is a "major unrecognized health problem."[198] It affects all people living in the northern hemisphere, including the northern United States, where sun exposure is inadequate for many months of the year.[199] Consequently, people in the North, when compared to those in the South, have more multiple sclerosis,[200] diabetes, rheumatoid arthritis,[201] osteoporosis,[202] hypertension,[203] cancer of the prostate,[204] cancer of the colon, and cancer of the breast.[205]

Vitamin D acts on cancer cells through a receptor (**VDR**), which is present in many types of cancer cells. A receptor is an usher molecule that helps hormones and other vital molecules do their work inside the cell. Via this receptor, vitamin D causes an arrest in the growth of cancer cells, makes them change back into normal cells (***differentiation***) and makes them commit suicide (***apoptosis***).[206] Vitamin D also blocks the effect of IGF-1 and estrogen receptor pathways in breast cancer cells.[207]

The cancer inhibitory effects of vitamin D are so significant that drug companies are now developing vitamin D ***analogs*** (synthetic brothers) to prevent and treat breast cancer.[208, 209] It is my belief that before we jump on to analogs, we should correct the widespread vitamin D deficiency in the Northern United States.

Concerns for skin beauty and skin cancer have made people avoid the sun by staying indoors or using increasingly potent sun blockers. The pendulum is swinging from sun worship to sun avoidance, an unhealthy trend, which will increase vitamin D deficiency and its associated diseases.

Dr. Michael Hollick advises his patients to go under the tanning bed for brief periods once a week or so in the winter. I agree with him. Just cover your face and neck and make sure to get out before you burn. That may mean: 5 to 8 minutes for fair skinned people, around 8 to 10 minutes for intermediate skin types, and 10 to15 minutes for African Americans. However, before you embark on this practice, clear it with your health care professional, making sure that you don’t have sun sensitivity or other contra-indications to UV exposure, and know your limits.

In summary, vitamin supplementation is preventive against breast cancer if used appropriately. In addition to a good multivitamin, natural (complete) vitamin E, folate (especially in women who drink alcohol), vitamin B12 (especially in menopausal women), and vitamin D (with supplementation or careful use of tanning beds in the winter), can help prevent breast cancer.

Chapter 22
Supplements for Breast Cancer Prevention

Supplements for breast cancer prevention carry a certain appeal. They provide an easy route to health and prevention, much easier than developing a regular exercise program or getting rid of body fat.

Many supplements have been talked about from time to time. Some make more sense than others; a few are backed by solid research, others, by hype. I have done a great deal of searching through the scientific literature, and over the years selected those that, I believe, have merit in the prevention of breast cancer.

In this chapter, I am going to discuss six supplements, starting with the ones that need a bit more research, and finishing with those that I believe are definitely helpful.

Selenium

Way back in 1969, when I was a resident in training, Professor Murray, from the University of Minnesota, made a trip to Hunza Valley, in the north of Pakistan, where people seem to live the longest. He found many 100-year olds still working in the fields, in spite of the fact that many of them smoked. There were few heart attacks, and virtually no cancer. When he came back, Professor Murray gave us a talk about the extraordinary longevity of the Hunzans. He thought that there were several reasons why these people lived so long; but the most impressive was the fact that they had "extremely high, almost toxic, levels of selenium in their blood."

Since then, I have read or heard many times that selenium is good for health, that it is a cancer preventive agent. Still, I find inconsistencies in the literature: some reports are positive, others show no benefit. For example, Finland increased the average intake of selenium in its population in 1984. By the year 2000, there had been "no significant effect" on the rate of cancer.[210] However, one cannot be certain that, without selenium, the cancer rates in Finland might have increased.

More recent work from the Institute of Cancer Prevention, American Health Foundation Cancer Center, Valhalla, NY, and elsewhere, suggests that one of the organic forms of selenium, ***Se-Methylselenocysteine,*** is a potent anti-cancer agent, preventing proliferation of breast cancer cells and making them commit suicide (apoptosis).[211, 212]

Most vitamin and mineral supplements have some selenium. I recommend that you use the ones that contain organic selenium.

Chrysin

Chrysin is a natural, plant derived substance, a ***flavone*** (also found in honey) that has been used by sportsmen and body builders to increase muscle mass and strength. I became aware of its mode of action some 10 years ago and have intermittently taken it myself.

Chrysin is a ***natural inhibitor of aromatase,*** the enzyme that converts androgens into estrogens, the very enzyme that has been implicated in the promotion of breast cancer. Studies since 1984 have shown chrysin to be quite potent in this respect.[213, 214]

A study from the Department of Food Science and Nutrition, University of Minnesota, compared a strong pharmaceutical aromatase inhibitor called ***aminoglutethamide (AG)*** with natural substances, using human fat cell cultures. They found that of the natural aromatase inhibitors, chrysin was the most potent, actually more potent than AG itself.[215]

During the last several years, my interest in chrysin has grown considerably. The reason is that synthetic aromatase inhibitors, such as Arimidex, Aromasin and Femara, are showing considerable anti-breast cancer effects and are being regularly employed to prevent recurrence in breast cancer patients. My thinking is: if synthetic stuff is showing results, what's wrong with using the real thing?

Unfortunately, there won't be any clinical research on chrysin, not any time soon. It is a natural substance that cannot be patented, and it is cheap. Pharmaceutical research has to focus on patentable compounds.

For now, I use it sparingly and intermittently, in women whom

I consider to be at high risk for breast cancer.

Mushroom Products

During the last 5 years, certain mushroom derivatives have been marketed heavily as anti-cancer agents. Most of the research behind their claims occurred in Japan, where some of the mushrooms have been served as delicacies for centuries, and where there is a general belief that these mushrooms are promoters of good health. Research on these products shows that, among other immune enhancing effects, there is an increase in the natural killer (NK) cell activity. Natural killer cells are our first defense against cancer cells. They are often impaired as a result of surgery, radiation therapy and chemotherapy. Hence the logic in stimulating them with mushrooms.

One such product, the "***Maitake fraction D***" of the Maitake mushroom, is marketed by Maitake Products, Inc. in Paramus, NJ. Most of the underlying research, on fraction D, was done by Kodama and Associates from the Department of Microbial Chemistry, Kobe Pharmaceutical University, Japan. They demonstrated that Maitake fraction D increased NK cell activity and ***IL-2*** (another cancer suppressive humor) in cancer patients[216] and decreased the spread of cancer in these patients.[217] They reported that "cancer regression or symptom improvement" occurred in many patients, including 68% of the patients with breast cancer.[218]

The second significant mushroom product is ***active hexose-correlated compound*** or ***AHCC***. It is being marketed under the trade name of ***ImmPower***, by American BioSciences, Inc. in Blauvlt, NY. Researchers in Osaka, Japan, have shown that AHCC increases IL-2 in tumor bearing mice,[219] and that it delays recurrence and prolongs survival in patients with liver cancer.[220]

These products are exciting, but expensive, and need a little more research. I am in favor of using them in patients who have already had breast cancer and are likely to have impaired immune function as a result of therapy. Routine use in all women does not appear justified until we have more experience with these substances.

Lycopene

Lycopene is a ***carotinoid*** (a relative of carotene) found in red and yellow fruits and vegetables, but particularly in tomatoes. In order to be digested and be absorbed into the system, it has to be mixed with fat, such as tomato sauce with fatty food. It cannot be absorbed by eating raw tomatoes. It is also available as a supplement in oily capsules.

The anti-cancer effects of lycopene have been known for some time. It is well known that it shrinks prostate cancer and improves outcomes in these patients. Its role in breast cancer also appears to be favorable.

A study from Ben-Gurion University of the Negev, Israel, reported in 1995, showed that lycopene was a potent inhibitor of human cancer cell proliferation.[221] It seems to do so by several mechanisms. For example, it has been shown to interfere with the growth promoting effect of IGF-1 on breast cancer cells.[222] It improves the expression of breast cancer suppressor genes, BRCA1 and BRCA2.[223] An enzyme called ***cyclin-dependent kinase*** promotes growth of cancer cells; lycopene reduces cyclin D in these cells, thereby diminishing this enzyme and cancer cell growth.[224]

Case control studies, however, have produced conflicting results. Some studies suggest that dietary intake of lycopene has no significant effect on the risk of breast cancer.[225, 226] Others, such as those from Umea University, Sweden, and Johns Hopkins, Maryland, reveal a significant protective effect.[227, 228]

Lycopene capsules are inexpensive. It is a natural substance, a carotenoid related to the vitamin A family, is found in many healthful foods, and can do no harm. I tend to give it to women whenever I sense a higher risk for breast cancer.

I3C (indole 3 carbinol)

In chapter 3, I discussed the cancer promoting effect of 16 alpha-hydroxyestrone, and in chapter 9 the preventive effect of 2-hydroxyestrone, both of these being metabolites (derivatives) of estradiol. I3C diminishes the former (16E) and increases the latter

(2E), thus inhibiting breast cancer. I3C is the active anti-breast cancer agent in ***cruciferous vegetables*** (broccoli, brussels sprouts, cauliflower, and cabbage). It has been purified and is available in capsules.

Further research with I3C has revealed that it has multiple anti-cancer activities. It decreases cyclin D, thus blocking the cancer cell cycle and its growth. I3C causes malignant cells to commit suicide (apoptosis)[229] while sparing normal breast cells.[230] It does so by blocking ***Nuclear Factor-kappa B*** in the cancer cells.[231]

I3C enhances the activity of BRCA1, the breast cancer suppressor gene, and stops the migration and invasion, or in other words, the spread of cancer cells.[232, 233] It is repressive to the estrogen receptor alpha (ER alpha), which is essential for the cancer promoting effect of estrogen.[234]

Cancer cells have a protein called ***MUCI,*** which helps them spread. The larger the amount of MUCI, the more aggressive the cancer becomes. I3C inhibits the formation of MUCI.[235] I3C stimulates the expression of ***Interferon gamma*** in the cancer cells, a substance that is naturally inhibitory to cancer cells.[236]

If there is any way breast cancer cells can be challenged and subdued, I3C knows that way. It is an amazing substance that nature has given us. And now, I3C is available as an affordable capsule, which easy to take. A 3 month study in normal women taking 400mg /day has demonstrated that it causes a sustained increase in 2-hydroxyestrone, without any side effects.[237] The cancer-preventive dose of I3C is 300-400 mg per day.[238]

I recommend I3C to many of my female patients, unless they have a known allergy to cruciferous vegetables.

Green Tea Extract (GTE)

Among the advanced nations in the world, the Japanese people, especially those from Okinawa, have the longest life spans. Many reasons have been cited for this longevity, but one of the most noted has to do with the consumption of green tea.

Dr.Kenichi Kitani, from the National Institute of Longevity Sciences, Tokyo Japan, participated in the American Academy of Anti-Aging Medicine in Las Vegas in 1995. After talking about anti-oxidants and other compounds, he concluded with the statement: "Despite the fact that my trip to Las Vegas has not been sponsored by any Japanese tea company, it is my suggestion that the answer to the question why Japanese can achieve a much longer life expectancy, may be their long traditional habit of drinking green tea." Dr. Kitani still believes in this statement, and has expressed his views in a recent article in the Annals of New York Academy of Sciences.[239]

How does green tea work against breast cancer? Let us look at the mechanisms and the evidence.

Back in 1993, researchers from the National Cancer Research Institute, Cancer Prevention Division, Tokyo, published an article on the anti-cancer activity of green tea.[240] They found that green tea extract—and its ingredients called ***catechins***- blocked the effect of estrogen on its receptor, reducing the growth of human breast cancer cells in culture dishes.

Other researchers demonstrated several additional mechanisms. It was found that GTE blocks the bad enzyme we have been talking about, aromatase,[241] and that it causes breast cancer cells to commit suicide (apoptosis) by blocking another enzyme called ***telomerase,*** which confers immortality upon cancer cells.[242] Furthermore, green tea reduces cyclin D, HER-2, BCL-2, and EGFR,[243] things which are beyond the scope of this book, but which all increase the growth and malignant potential of breast cancer cells.

In addition, green tea has been shown to inhibit ***fatty acid synthase*** (FAS), which leads to proliferation of cancer cells.[244] It blocks the "***angiogenic fibroblast growth factor,***" which promotes the growth of blood vessels inside tumors.[245] Blood vessels feed tumors, causing growth and helping cancer cells spread to other parts of the body.

Another factor that grows blood vessels is called the ***vascular endothelial growth factor*** (**VEGF**). GTE suppresses this factor too.[246]

A gene called ***p21*** protects us against cancer. It is a 'tumor suppressor gene.' GTE enhances the function of this gene.[247]

What about human studies? Although some authors suggest that green tea consumption has no significant effect on breast cancer,[248] the preponderance of scientific evidence points to a major anti-cancer effect.

Dr. Nakachi from the Department of Epidemiology, Radiation Effects Research Foundation, Hiroshima, Japan (the site of nuclear bombing), in a 13-year follow up of people, found that green tea consumption delayed cancer onset and all-cause mortality in these Japanese populations.[249]

Many investigators have shown that human breast cancers grown in animals are suppressed by GTE .[250, 251]

Others have shown that green tea consumption decreases the recurrence rate in patients who already have stage I or II breast cancer and are in remission.[252, 253]

Dr. A.H. Wu and associates from the Department of Preventive Medicine, University of Southern California, School of Medicine, LA, interviewed Chinese, Japanese and Filipino women in LA county. They compared 501 of these women who had breast cancer with 594 who did not. Women who drank green tea had significantly less cancer than those who did not. The greater the amount of green tea ingested, the higher the degree of protection was observed.[254]

So, here is another gift from nature. There is overwhelming evidence that green tea is not only responsible in decreasing cancer, but also decreases overall mortality, including that from heart disease. If it were a drug, you can be certain it would be quite expensive. Yet it is available in a pure, natural and effective form in a capsule, for around $ 10 a bottle. All evidence suggests that it is health promoting and a breast cancer antagonist and that it has no side effects. Volunteers who took 15 tablets per day for 6 months had absolutely no side effects.[255] An average tablet or capsule is the equivalent of drinking almost 5 cups of green tea.

I put all my women patients on green tea extract.

Chapter 23
Anti-inflammatory Drugs (Aspirin, Ibuprofen, Celebrex, etc.)

Taking any drug on a long-term basis worries me. Modern day drugs (pharmaceuticals) are, for the most part, compounds that are foreign to our bodies. In order to improve a problem at hand — such as lowering cholesterol or blood pressure, or reducing arthritis pain — they block an enzyme here, or subdue a receptor there; but they can have far- reaching and hidden effects on the cell's chemistry and machinery, effects that take years to emerge . . . and that can hurt us in the end.

It has been estimated that more than 100,000 Americans die each year as a result of these side effects. That is more than twice the number who die from breast cancer. Yet there are drugs that have stood the test of time, drugs whose benefits and side effects are well known, and whose benefits outweigh the side effects when used appropriately.

Aspirin is one such drug. In chapter 6, I discussed the role of silent inflammation in the causation of many chronic diseases, including cancer. Aspirin and other anti-inflammatory drugs reduce inflammation. Let me explain how it all works.

The main culprit in the inflammatory process is the enzyme ***COX-2***, which:

- turns on the aromatase gene, thus making more estrogen,
- impairs p53, a tumor suppressor gene,
- turns on several ***oncogenes*** or tumor promoting genes, including HER-2, which makes breast cancer more aggressive,
- increases Bcl-2 protein, which prevents apoptosis (cancer cell suicide),
- promotes several "***angiogenesis***" factors, which grow new blood vessels in and around the tumor to facilitate its growth and spread.[256]

COX-2 levels have been found to be increased in breast cancer tissue. Dr. C. Denkert, from the Institute of Pathology, Charite Hospital, Berlin, Germany, analyzed 8 different studies compiling 2392 cases of breast cancer. Forty percent of all these cancers were found to be positive for COX-2.[257]

Aspirin and other anti-inflammatory drugs can be valuable because they work against COX-2.

Some studies have shown that regular users of aspirin have 30% less breast cancer than non-users.[258] Other studies looking at the collective use of all of these anti-inflammatory drugs reveal that the protection may even be higher, as much as 40 to 50%.[259, 260] In addition, the breast cancers that do develop in these patients tend to be smaller, have less involvement of the lymph nodes, and are, therefore, more curable.

A recent study from the Division of Breast Surgery, University of Hong Kong Medical Centre, used aromatase inhibitors with or without Celebrex in the treatment of breast cancer. Complete remissions were only seen in the group that included Celebrex.[261]

This is the reason why drug companies and various cancer centers across the world are launching clinical studies on the use of COX-2 inhibitors (particularly Celebrex) in the prevention of breast cancer.[262]

So, what is the reader to do? Start taking these drugs? For the moment, I believe we should use caution.

Vioxx , Celabrex, and other COX-2 inhibitors have resulted in heart attacks and strokes in this country and have been withdrawn from the market. Personally, I would not put patients on modern COX-2 inhibitors on a long term basis.

On the other hand, aspirin is a very old drug. We have known it for a very long time. I have advised a baby aspirin to hundreds of patients at high risk for a heart attack. I do the same for women who are overweight and have a high ***CRP*** (C reactive protein), indicating that they have silent inflammation. I just make sure that they don't have a tendency towards stomach problems. It is interesting to note that the National Institute on Aging (NIA) is studying the effect of lifelong administration of small doses of aspirin on the life span. I have a feeling that it will reveal benefit in participants with high CRP levels. Benefit in a large population, without regard to CRP, is difficult to predict.

Other anti-inflammatory drugs, such as 'statins' used for high cholesterol, may show a similar anti-cancer effect in the future. Currently, some research is being conducted in this area.

In the end, I feel that all such use of drugs should be under the care of a qualified physician, who can evaluate the risks and benefits in any given patient.

Chapter 24
Stress Reduction

This book would be incomplete without saying a word or two about stress and its possible relationship with breast cancer. Stress and breast cancer have been connected since biblical times. We have all heard about women developing breast cancer after a major personal loss or depression. I have personally seen women like this in my practice.

The National Cancer Institute's position is that there is no definitive proof that stress leads to breast cancer. The studies showing such association have had "flaws."[263, 264]

However, it is an established fact that stress and depression can inhibit our immune system, our T cells and natural killer cells, which are important in our defense against cancer.[265]

A recent study from the Iranian Center for Breast Cancer, Tehran, has revealed a distinct relationship between depression and feelings of hopelessness and subsequent development of breast cancer.[266] Over a period of 3 years, 3,000 women came to the center and were interviewed in detail about all possible factors related to breast cancer, including stress and depression. Subsequently, 243 of these women were found to have breast cancer. When compared to those who were did not have cancer, breast cancer patients had had significantly more "prior depressed mood and feelings of hopelessness."

Another group of researchers surveyed 1213 women from the Baltimore area, including 29 who developed breast cancer over the years.[267] They found that maternal death or severe episodes of depression 20 years before the onset of cancer significantly increased the chance of cancer in these women. Relatively recent life events, anxiety or depression did not have any impact.

Stress permeates the world community and its level seems to be rising every day. There is no question that it affects health in many ways – a possibly higher breast cancer risk being just one. We need to make an effort to reduce stress, not by taking anti-depressants (whose use is sky-rocketing in America), but by using more natural techniques such as deep breathing, meditation, yoga, exercise and our own personal spirituality.

- Section 4 -
Guidelines to Stop Breast Cancer

Chapter 25
The Breast Cancer Prevention Guidelines

Knowing how breast cancer starts, how it grows and spreads, and the various factors that promote or inhibit this growth, can help one assemble a guideline for its prevention. We may not be able to entirely prevent breast cancer, but we can delay its appearance by years, reduce suffering and expense, and make a real difference in the quality of a woman's life.

The following is an outline of my system. It does not fit every woman precisely. It differs from woman to woman, depending on age, menopausal status, risk factors and whether or not she has had breast cancer previously. Other minor factors often come into play, so I find myself bending and shaping the guideline to fit every woman. It is a guideline that can help you to stave off breast cancer. It is not something that can replace your own physician's advice and care, which is based on your own unique health history and clinical condition.

General Guideline for all Women

1. Exercise

There is no question that regular exercise reduces the risk of breast cancer by about 25%, as well as the risk of most other diseases.

The key question is: why do 70% of Americans neglect to exercise? There is no clear-cut answer. It depends on the personality type, amount of motivation, domestic, social and financial circumstances, and quite frequently, on plain-old lack of energy. I find that when I can pinpoint the reason for lack of energy and correct it, and create an exercise program that fits individual circumstances, most women frequently begin to exercise. Even then, there are road blocks and hurdles. But for a physician to simply say to a patient "go exercise" is an exercise in futility. It almost never works.

Healthy exercise does not have to be extreme. Actually, severe exercise generates a lot of free radicals and may even depress the immune system. Moderate exercise seems to be the ticket. It has to include some warm up, some strength training and a 20 to 30 minute aerobic component (see chapter 18), 3 to 4 times each week. In addition, I feel it is necessary to have what I call "mini-bursts" of activity throughout the day, whenever you can think of them. These mini bursts may be different things to different people, like climbing stairs, walking briskly while shopping, moving stuff around the house, a quick walk before lunch, 5 to10 minutes on the treadmill any time of the day, doing a few push ups against your desk, a few lunges in the hall – in fact any such activity you can think of. The idea is to keep your metabolic rate up as much as possible throughout the day. If you sit at a desk all day, your metabolic rate will drop and remain low all day. Moderate exercise 3 times a week by itself will not maintain a higher metabolic rate the entire week. Mini bursts will do so. I have seen many patients who lose 10 lbs with this technique, and some who have lost up to 25 lbs. Such loss – of fat only, while improving muscle tone and mass – should be the real objective. Quick weight loss with gimmicks is unhealthy; it always returns, with more body fat and less muscle mass.

2. Food

What to eat

- Start your day with a ***protein*** rich breakfast such as a 3 to 4 egg-white omelet with veggies (include one omega-3 egg yoke), or a whey protein powder shake with some berries and 1 to 2% milk (milk fat is not bad), or a piece of salmon, cottage cheese, or even a few links of sausage occasionally. Keep toast and refined cereal to a minimum. Think protein at breakfast. If you start out right you will end the day right. Protein will increase your metabolic rate, induce a healthy release of human growth hormone, increase your anti-inflammatory prostaglandins, keep your insulin level low and prevent you from getting hungry. A carbohydrate breakfast will move everything in the opposite direction. Besides, you will be hungry before noon, and need more carbohydrates. Carbohydrates will throw you into a vicious carbohydrate cycle.

- ***Vegetables and fruits*** are important. Use only organic produce to exclude pesticides. Focus on the cruciferous vegetables (broccoli, Brussels sprouts, cabbage, cauliflower). They contain I3C which changes estrogen into 2-hydroxyestrone, the 'good' estrogen. Keep very sweet fruits (bananas, pineapple) to a minimum. They will raise your insulin level.
- Think ***fiber*** (fruits, veggies, whole grain products). Fiber will bind toxins and estrogen as they drip into the intestine, and remove them from your body.
- Keep red meat (saturated) ***fats*** to a minimum. Avoid any hydrogenated or partially hydrogenated fats, which stiffen the walls of your cells and blunt insulin receptors, thus increasing insulin resistance. If using vegetable oils, include protein with them to increase PG-1 (anti-inflammatory) as much as possible. Do not heat the oil for a long time (to prevent oxidation, which will release free radicals in the system). Exclude any rancid oil, for the same reason. Foods like French fries will increase free radicals (from overheated oxidized oil), increase insulin (from the refined carbohydrate), and increase PG-2 (by combining carbohydrate with omega-6 oil), thus increasing inflammation in your body . . . all the wrong things! Increase omega-3 fats that are found in walnuts and flax seed, but more importantly in deep sea fish such as wild salmon. Avoid farmed fish, which generally has a high content of dioxins, mercury and other chemicals. Supplement with good quality fish oil capsules, making

sure that these are guaranteed to be free of mercury, dioxins and other toxins. Use liberal quantities of high quality olive oil (omega-9).

- Get rid of ***sugar and refined (white) starches***, as much as possible.
- Keep ***alcohol*** intake to a minimum. Red wine is a better choice, because it is full of anti-oxidants, it is an aromatase inhibitor and it has reserveratrol, which has anti-cancer activity.

How to Eat

- ***Take your time.*** Eat slowly, while thoroughly chewing your food. This will help you digest your food better and know when you are getting full. If you eat fast, your brain does not register when you are full. As a rule, the faster you eat the bigger your waistline will be.
- Cultural habits (not getting up from the table before finishing your plate, drinking giant colas, eating large fast-food portions) I believe, have increased the capacity of the American stomach. We have an extra large tank. I think we can shrink it, if we leave a little space in it every time we eat, and bring it back to a reasonable size. ***Do not eat until you are full;*** make it a habit.

When to eat

- Eat three meals a day and ***avoid snacks,*** especially carbohydrate snacks. Normally, after a meal your body releases insulin and disposes of carbohydrates for approximately 3 hours. Then it shifts gear and begins to burn fat, which is extremely important to maintain a healthy body composition. A snack 2 to 3 hours after your meal will stop this important change because now your body has to release insulin again. You will be constantly struggling, burning carbohydrates, and not getting rid of the extra fat in your body. This is especially true of the late night snacks like the popcorn with the10 PM news! You can learn to avoid such snacks if you focus on protein at every meal. You won't be as hungry in 3 hours. Dieticians often advise patients to eat snacks in between meals. I believe this approach can only work if the main meals are very small with small amounts of carbohydrates. The way most people eat they cannot afford to add snacks and still burn fat. If you have to have something, try a few nuts — just a few.

3. Vitamins and minerals

- ***Multivitamin and mineral supplements*** should be a must for everyone. Talk to a nutritionist or other health-care professional to select the best kind for you.
- ***Vitamin E*** preparations should be natural and complete. Avoid the alpha tocopherol-only preparations that have been commonly sold to the public. They deplete the body of the important vitamin E, gamma tocopherol, which has anti-cancer and anti-heart disease activity. Several companies are beginning to make such preparations and giving them different names, such as High E, Perfect E, etc.
- ***Folic acid*** 600 micrograms a day is a must, especially for women who drink alcohol.
- ***Vitamin D*** deficiency is prevalent in the northern states and other northern countries, because of lack of exposure to the UV-B lights of the sun. Ordinary supplements are insufficient and cannot make up for the natural mechanism, sun exposure, for making the necessary supply of this important vitamin. Beside other health benefits, vitamin D fights breast cancer in several different ways. Select a vitamin D and calcium supplement that provides 800 IUs of vitamin D/day. If you live in the northern hemisphere with reduced sun exposure six months out of a year, consider short exposures to UV-B lights in a tanning booth once every week or two in the winter. Cover your face and neck with a towel, and get out before burning. It should be a short

exposure: 5-8 minutes for fair skinned people, 8-10 minutes for intermediate types and 10-15 minutes for African Americans. Make sure you don't have a contra-indication to UV exposure, by talking to your health care provider. This suggestion may seem odd to many people. However, vitamin D deficiency is the cause of many serious health problems, which cannot be ignored. If you can travel to a warm sunny spot for long weekends several times a winter, that is the best solution; you won't have the need for tanning beds. And it will help with stress reduction to boot!

4. Supplements

- ***Green Tea Extract.*** It is my belief that all women should be taking GTE, unless they have some kind of an allergy or sensitivity to this important supplement. As I have explained, GTE fights breast cancer in numerous ways, and has other healthful effects. It is one of the reasons why Okinawans live so long.

5. Breast and Nipple Stimulation

- There are no clinical studies to prove the benefits of this practice; but there is scientific evidence that it increases the secretion of oxytocin, which not only helps remove pent-up secretions from the breast ducts, but also fights breast cancer in several ways. Besides, it reduces stress. Such practice should be hygienic and non-traumatic.

Additional Guidelines

Ages 20 to 30

- ***Breast feed,*** as long as possible. Your baby will be healthier and will have a higher IQ. You will be healthier; more relaxed and have less breast cancer.
- Keep ***birth control pill*** use to a minimum. It increases the risk of breast cancer slightly.
- If you have ***infertility problems,*** have your progesterone levels checked. If your progesterone level is consistently low, you are at a future risk for breast cancer. It should be watched and controlled by someone who understands ***natural bio-identical hormones***. Progesterone should never be replaced by 'progestin' or 'progestagen,' the artificial-synthetic and harmful 'hormones.'

Ages 30 to 45

- If you have a great deal of **PMS,** you very likely have estrogen dominance and/or progesterone insufficiency, which needs to be diagnosed with appropriate testing. You may have bloating, breast tenderness, irritability, anxiety, depression or even panic attacks. Prolonged estrogen dominance will increase your risk of breast cancer. Do not just go on an anti-depressant. Seek a health care professional who knows the correct use of natural bio-identical hormones. Appropriate doses of natural progesterone to balance your hormones may be all you need.
- If there is a **family history of breast cancer** (mother, aunts and siblings), consider getting genetic testing for BRCA 1 and II gene abnormalities.
- If you are gaining too much weight, especially around the abdomen, it is a sign of **insulin resistance**, which leads to all types of health problems including breast cancer. You may need to have several things checked such as fasting insulin level, blood sugar, CRP, SHBG (sex hormone binding globulin), estrogen, progesterone, testosterone, etc. You should seek a health care professional who focuses on ***prevention***, and who understands natural bio-identical

hormones. A *board* certified anti-aging specialist will be the most appropriate for this task. Look for one in your area. Based on the above, if your risk of breast cancer is judged to be higher than normal, consider adding ***indole 3 carbinol (I3C)*** to your supplements.

- If you have cold intolerance (hands and feet are cold, or "freezing all the time"), dry skin, thinning coarse hair, weight gain and rising cholesterol (symptoms suggesting low thyroid) make sure to have your free T3 and other thyroid tests checked. If you free T3 is low or at the lower end of normal, you may benefit from a low dose of Armour thyroid. Discuss it with your doctor or consult an anti-aging specialist.

Ages 45 and above

- Ages 30 to 45 guidelines may apply to women in this age group
- If you are having any hormonal symptoms such as ***hot flashes, night sweats, trouble sleeping, brain fog, vaginal dryness, lack of muscle tone, low libido, etc.***, see a physician who understands natural bio-identical hormones. This will be your best bet. Avoid artificial and synthetic hormones. Even natural hormones may increase your risk if given inappropriately. You need to have your hormones measured and increased only as necessary. Several of these hormones are safer if given as skin creams to avoid passage through the liver and the so called "first pass liver effect" which can result in certain complications. Again, seek a health care professional who is experienced and understands the use of these hormones.
- You may need to have ***additional hormones*** such as DHEA, human growth hormones, etc., checked and managed appropriately. Indiscriminate use of these hormones is unhealthy. They should be used only if necessary, with caution and never in large amounts. Too much of a good thing is always bad.
- ***Excess weight, insulin resistance and inflammation (high CRP)*** are common problems in this age group and need to be managed appropriately. With

increased CRP, one baby aspirin/day would help reduce the risk of breast cancer among other benefits.

- ***Additional supplements*** such as ***lycopene*** can be added at this time. In over- weight women with large breasts and relatively high estrogen levels, it may be appropriate to add ***chrysin*** as a supplement. It is a natural aromatase inhibitor and will reduce the formation of estrogen in the fat cells of the breast. I use chrysin intermittently, and focus more on reducing body fat.
- ***If you are having trouble sleeping,*** consider adding melatonin, the smallest effective dose, 1 hour before bedtime, 3 to 4 times a week. Even if it does not improve your sleep, it has anti-cancer effects and many other benefits.

Women with a history of previous breast cancer

- ***General guidelines*** will be of help to all women including those with history of previous breast cancer
- ***Excess weight, insulin resistance and inflammation*** should be managed rigorously. This should be under the care of a knowledgeable health care professional. Body fat should be reduced, SHBG increased, fasting insulin should be lowered and inflammation should be cut down as much as possible.
- ***Supplements*** should include green tea extract, indole 3 carbinol and lycopene. Chrysin should be considered for women with excess body fat. Women with diminished immune response after chemo and radiation would very likely benefit from the mushroom supplements. Melatonin 3 to 4 nights per week would be a useful addition for all such women.
- ***Hormonal therapy*** for menopausal women with a history of breast cancer has been avoided by conventional medicine. However, there is evidence that in patients who have remained free of cancer for five years, estrogen therapy does not increase the rate of recurrence. If at all, there is a suggestion that such patients have less recurrence (see chapter 4). As an oncologist and an anti-aging

physician with considerable experience in each field, it is my belief that withholding hormonal therapy in this situation would be detrimental to the health of many such women. For patients who have remained free of cancer for five years, hormonal therapy should be considered if they have: impaired quality of life, osteoporosis, or risk factors for cardiovascular disease or Alzheimer's disease. If the decision is made to institute such therapy, it should consist of natural estriol (with or without small amounts of estradiol), progesterone and testosterone. Oral estrogen should be avoided, as it increases CRP, an inflammatory state. Hormone levels should be monitored and kept at modest levels, while avoiding breast tenderness (an estrogenic effect). Again, you will need to work with a physician who is experienced and knowledgeable in this field, who understands breast cancer and the use of natural bio-identical hormones.

I hope that these guidelines will fulfill the particular needs of most, if not all, women. These guidelines are as comprehensive as possible in light of the current scientific knowledge, but they will evolve with time as more knowledge accumulates. It is my hope that most physicians will offer such advice and guidelines to their patients. Too many women are dying, suffering or losing quality of life as a result of breast cancer. Let us make an effort to stop it.

References

1. Proceedings of the American Society of Clinical Oncology, 2003
2. Proceedings of the American Society of Clinical Oncology, 2004
3. Chen G, Djuric Z. Detection of 2,6 cyclolycopene-I,5-diol in breast nipple aspirate fluids and plasma: a potential marker of oxidative stress. Cancer Epidemiol Biomarkers Prev. 2002 Dec; 11(12): 1592-6
4. Murrell TG Epidemiological and biochemical support for a theory on the cause and prevention of breast cancer. Med Hypotheses 1991 Dec; 36(4):389-96
5. Collaborative group on hormonal factors in breast cancer. Breast cancer and breast feeding: collaborative reanalysis of individual data from 47 epidemiological studies in 30 countries. Lancet 2002 Jul 20; 360(9328)187-95
6. Jefcoate CR et al. Tissue-specific synthesis and oxidative metabolism of estrogens. J Natl Cancer Inst Monogf.2000;(27):95-112
7. Chang M, et al. Inhibition of glutathione S transferase activity by the quinoid metabolites of equine estrogens. Chem Tes Toxicol. 1998 Jul;11(7):758-65
8. Jhanwar-Uniyal M. BRCA 1 in cancer ,cell cycle and genomic stability. Front Biosci. 2003 SEP 1;8:S1107-17
9. World cancer research fund panel (Potter JD chair). Food, nutrition and the prevention of cancer; a global perspective. Washington, DC: American Institute for Cancer Research, 1997
10. Wattenberg L. Chemoprevention of cancer. Cancer Res. 1985; 45:1-8
11. Wattenberg L. Inhibition of neoplasia by minor dietary constituents. Cancer Res 1983; 43: 2448s-2448s
12. Weisburger JH. Antimutagens, anticarcinogens and effective world wide cancer prevention. J Environ Pathol Toxicol Oncol. 1999;18(2):85-93
13. Smith-Warner SA, et al. Intake of fruits and vegetables and risk of breast cancer. JAMA 2001;285:769-76
14. Friedenreich CM. Review of anthropometric factors and breast cancer risk. Eur J Cancer Prev 2001; 10:15-32
15. Murrell TG. The potential for oxytocin to prevent breast cancer: a hypothesis. Breast Cancer Res Treat 1995; 35(2):225-9
16. Coiro V, et al. Inhibition by ethanol of the oxytocin response to breast stimulation in normal women and the role of endogenous opioids. Acta Endocrinol (Copenh) 1992Mar;126(3):213-6

17. 3.Friberg S, Mattson S. On the growth rates of human malignant tumors: implications for medical decision making. J Surg Oncol. 1997 Aug; 65(4)284-97

18. 4.Kuroishi T, et al. Tumor growth rate and prognosis of breast cancer mainly detected by mass screening. Jpn J Cancer Res. 1990 May; 81(5):454-62

19. Mendelsohn ME. Protective effects of estrogens on the cardiovascular system. Am J Cardiol 2002 jun 20; 89(12 supplement):12-7

20. McEwen B. The molecular and neuroanatomical basis of estrogen effects in the central nervous system. J Clin Endocrinol Metab.1999;84:1790-97

21. Key TJ. Serum oestradiol and breast cancer risk. Endocr Relat Cancer. 1999 Jun;6(2):175-80

22. Key TJ et al. A prospective study of urinary oestrogen excretion and breast cancer risk. Br J Cancer. 1996 Jun;73(12)1615-9

23. Mady EA, etal. Sex steroid hormones in serum and breast tissue of benign and malignant breast tumor patients. Dis Markers. 2000;16(304):151-7

24. Pasqualini JR, et al. Importance of estrogen sulfates in breast cancer. J Steroid Biochem. 1989;34(1-6):155-63

25. Jefcoate CR, et al. Tissue-specific synthesis and oxidative metabolism of estrogens. J Natl Cancer Inst Monogr. 2000;(27):95-112

26. Brueggemeier RW, et al. Aromatase and cyclooxygenases: enzymes in breast cancer. J Steroid Biochem Mol Biol. 2003 Sep;86(3-5):501-7

27. Chelbowski RT, et al. Influence of estrogen plus progestin on hreast cancer and mammography in healthy post-menopausal women. The women's health initiative randomized trial. JAMA Jun 25.289(24):3243-53

28. Jernstrom H, et al. A prospective study of different types of hormone replacement therapy use and the risk of breast cancer: the women's health in the Lund area (WHILA) study (Sweden). Cancer Causes Control.2003 Sep;14(7):673080

29. Schairer C, et al. Cause-specific mortality in women receiving hormone replacement therapy. Epedemiology 1997 Jan;8(1):59-65

30. Vassilopoulou-Sellin R, et al. Estrogen replacement therapy after localized breast cancer. Clinical outcome of 319 women followed prospectively. J Clin Oncol 1999 May;17(5):1482-7

31. health in the Lund area (WHILA) study (Sweden). Cancer Causes Control.2003 Sep;14(7):673080

32. Kabat GC, et al. Urinary estrogen metabolites and breast cancer: a case control study. Cancer Epidemiol Biomarkers Prev. 1998 Jul;

6(7):505-9
33. Ursin G, et al. Urinary 2-hydroxyestrone/16 alpha-hydroxyestrone ratio and the risk of breast cancer in post-menopausal women. J Natl Cancer Inst. 1999 Jun 16;91(12):1067-72
34. .Longcope C, et al. The effect of a low fat diet on estrogen metabolism. J Clin Endocrinol Metab. 1987 Jun;64(6):1246-50
35. Starek A. Estrogens and organochlorine xenoestrogens and breast cancer risk. Int J Occup Med Environ Health. 2003;16(2):113-24
36. Dreher D, Junod, AF. Role of oxygen free radicals in cancer development. Eur J Cancer; 1996 Jan;32A(1):30-8
37. Athar M. Oxidative stress and experimental carcinogenesis. Indian J Exp Bio. 2002 Jun; 40(6):656-67
38. Morgan C, et al. Detection of p53 mutations in precancerous gastric tissue. Br J Cancer. 2003 Oct 6;89(7):1314-9
39. Hussain SP, et al. Oxy-radical induced mutagenesis of hotspot codons 248-249 of human p53 gene. Oncogene. 1994;9(8):2277-81
40. Gopalakrishna R, Jaken S. Protein kinase C signaling and oxidative stress. Free Radic Biol Med. 2000 May 1;28(9):1349-61
41. Ueji M, et al. Risk factors for breast cancer among Japanese women: A case-control study. Breast Cancer. 1998 Oct 25;5(4):351-58
42. Boyd DB. Insulin and Cancer. Integr Cancer Ther. 2003 Dec;2(4):315-29
43. Malin A, et al. Evaluation of the synergistic effect of insulin resistance and the insulin-like growth factors on the risk of breast carcinoma. Cancer. 2004 Feb 15; 100(4):694-700
44. Goodwin PJ, et al. Fasting Insulin and outcome in early-stage breast cancer: results of a prospective cohort study. Journal of Clinical Oncology 2002 Jan;20(1):42-51
45. Hankinson SE, et al. Circulating concentrations of IGF-1 and the risk of breast cancer. Lancet. 1998 May;351(9113):1393-96
46. Renehan AG, et al. Insulin like growth factor (IGF-1), IGF binding protein-3 and cancer risk:systematic review and meta-regression analysis. Lancet. 2004 April:363 (9418):1346-53
47. Michels KB, et al. Type 2 diabetes and subsequent incidence of breast cancer in the nurses' health study. Diabetes Care. 2003 26:1752-58
48. Simopoulos AP. The importance of the ratio of omega-6/omega-3 essential fatty acids. Biomed Pharmacother.2002 Oct;56(8):365-79
49. Karuppu D, et al. Aromatase and prostaglandin inter-relationships in breast adipose tissue: significance for breast cancer development. Breast Cancer Res Treat. 2002 Nov;76(2):103-9
50. Holmes MD, et al. Meta-analysis: dietary fat intake, serum estrogen

levels, and the risk of breast cancer. J Natl Cancer Inst 1999;91:1511-12

51. World Cancer research Fund Panel (Potter JD Chair). Food, nutrition and the prevention of cancer: a Global Perspective. Washington DC: American Institute for Cancer Research, 1997

52. Welsch CW. Relationship between dietary fat and animal mammary tumorogenesis: a review and critique. Cancer Res 1992;52(suppl 7)2040-48

53. Bartsch H, et al. Dietary polyunsaturated fatty acids and cancers of the breast and colorectum: emerging evidence for their role as risk modifiers. Cacinogenisis.1999 Dec;20(12):2209-18

54. Jandacek RL, Tso P. Factors affecting the storage and excretion of toxic lipohilic xenobiotics. Lipids. 2001 Dec;361(12):1289-305

55. Cottam DR, et al. The chronic inflammatory hypothesis for the morbidity associated with morbid obesity: implications and effects of weight loss. Obes Surg. 2004 May; 14(5):589-600

56. Rose DP, et al. Adverse effects of obesity on breast cancer prognosis, and the biological actions of leptin (review). Int J oncol. 2002 Dec;21(6):1285-92

57. Zumoff B. Hormonal abnormalities in obesity. Acta Med Scand Suppl. 1988;723:153-60

58. NcTiernan A. Behavioral risk factors in breast cancer: Can risk be modified? The Oncologist. 2003;8:326-334

59. Stoll BA. Teenage obesity in relation to breast cancer risk. Intl J obes Relat Metab Disord. 1998 Nov;221(11)1035-40

60. Singletary KW, et al. Alcohol and breast cancer: review of epidemiologic and experimental evidence and potential mechanisms. JAMA 2001;87:2143-51

61. Hamajima N, et al. Alcohol, tobacco and breast cancer-collaborative reanalysis of individual data from 53 epidemiological studies, including 58,515 women with breast cancer and 95,063 women without the disease. Br J Cancer 2002;87:1234-45

62. Etique N, et al. Ethanol stimulates proliferation , ERalpha and aromatase expression inn MCF-7 buman breast cancer cells. Int J Mol Med. 2004 Jan;13(1):149-55

63. Purohit V. Can alcohol promote aromatization of androgens ot estrogens? A review. Alcohol. 2000 Nov;22(3):123-7

64. Ginsburg ES, et al. Effects of alcohol ingestion on estrogens in post-menopausal women. JAMA. 1996 Dec 4;276(21):1747-51

65. Singletary KW, Gapstur SM. Alcohol and breast cancer: review of epidemiologic and experimental evidence and potential mechanisms. JAMA; 2001 Nov 7;286(17):2143-51

66. Poschl G, Seitz HK. Alcohol and cancer. Alcohol Alcohol.2004

May-Jun;39(3):155-65
67. Kalant H. Direct effects of ethanol on the nervous system. Fed Proc.1975 Sep;34(10):1930-41
68. Gunzerath L, et al. National Instiitue on Alcohol Abuse and Alcoholism report on moderate drinking. Alcohol Clin Exp Res. 2004 Jun;28(6):829-47
69. Eng ET, et al. Anti-aromatase chemicals in red wine. Ann NY Acad Sci. 2002 Jun;963:239-46
70. Lemon HM, et al. Reduced estriol excretion in patients with breast cancer prior to endocrine therapy. JAMA.1966;196:112-20
71. Lemon HM. Oestriol and prevention of breast cancer. The Lancet. 1973 March 10: 546-47
72. Lemon HM. Pathophysilogic considerations in the treatment of menopausal patients with oestrogens; the role of oestriol in the prevention of mammary carcinoma. Acta Endocrino Suppl (copenh) 1980;233:17-27
73. Siiteri PK. Pregnancy hormone estriol may reduce risk for breast cancer. Doctor's Guide 2002 Sept 30: www.pslgroup.com/
74. Bradlow HL, et al. 2-hydroxyestone: the 'good' estrogen. J Endocrinl. 1996 Sep;150 suppl:S259-65
75. Muti P, et al. Estrogen metabolism and the risk of breast cancer: a prospective study of the 2:16alpha-hydroxyestrone ratio in premenopausal and post menopausal women.
76. Jatoi I, et al. Timing of surgery for primary breast cancer with regard to the menstrual phase and prognosis. Breast Cancer Res Treat. 1998;52(1-3):217-25
77. Cowan LD, et al. Breast cancer incidence in women with a history of progesterone deficiency. Am J Epidemol. 1981;114(2):209-17
78. Formby B, Wiley TS. Progesterone inhibits growth and induces apoptosis in breast cancer cells: inverse effects on Bcl-2 and p53. Ann Clin Lab Sci. 1998 Nov-Dec;28(6):360-9
79. Formby B, wiley TS. Bcl-2, surviving and variant CD44 v7-v10 are downregulated and p53 is upregulated in breast cancer cells by progesterone: inhibition of cell growth and apoptosis. Mol Cell Biochem; 1999 Dec;202(1-2):53-61
80. Horita K, et al. Progesterone induces apoptosis in malignant melanoma cells. Anticancer Res; 2001 Nov-Dec;21(6A):3871-4
81. Sorensen MB, et al. Long-term use of contraceptive depot medroxyprogesterone acetate in young women impairs arterial endothelial function assessed by cardiovascular magnetic resonance. Circulation 2002 Sep 24;106(13):1646-51
82. Rosano GM, et al. Natural progesterone, but not

medroxyprogesterone acetate, enhances the beneficial effect of estrogen on exercise induced myocardial ischemia in postmenopausal women. J Am Coll Cardiol.2000 Dec;36(7):2154-9

83. Clarkson TB. Progestogens and cardiovascular disease. A critical review. J Reprod Med. 1999 Feb;44(2Suppl):180-4

84. Kahn HS, et al. Effects of injectable or implantable progestin-only contraceptioves on insulin-glucose metabolism and diabetes risk. Diabetes Care.2003 Jan;26(1):216-25

85. Sutherland RL, et al. Effects of medroxyprogesterone acetate on proliferation and cell cycle kinetics of human mammary carcinoma cells. Cancer Res. 1988 Sep 15;48(18):5084-91

86. Fournier A, et al. Breast cancer risk in relation to different types of hormone replacement therapy in the E3N-EPIC cohort. Int J Cancer. 2005 Apr 10;114(3):448-54

87. Lesnikov VA, Pierpaoli W. Pineal cross-transplantation (old-to-young and vice versa) as evidence for an endogenous "aging clock"Ann N Y Acad Sci. 1994 May 31; 719:456-60

88. Pieroaoli W. Lesnikov V. Theoretical considerations on the nature of the pineal 'ageing clock.' Genrontology. 1997;43(1-2):20-5

89. Pierpaoli W. Neuroimmunomodulation of aging. Aprogram in the pineal gland. Ann N Y Acad Sci. 1998 May 1;840:491-7

90. Coleman MP, Reiter RJ. Breast cancer, blindness and melatonin. Eur J Cancer. 1992;28(2-3):501-3

91. Anisimov VN. The light-dark regimen and cancer development. Neuro Endocrino Lett. 2002 Jul;23Suppl 2:28-36

92. Panzer A, Viljoen M. The validity of melatonin as an oncostatic agent. J Pineal Res. 1997 May;22(4):184-202

93. Sanchez-Barcelo EJ, et al. Melatonin and mammary cancer: a short review. Endocr Relat Cancer. 2003 Jun;10(2):153-9

94. Blask DE, et al. New actions of melatonin on tumor metabolism and growth. Biol Signals Recept. 1999 Jan-Apr;8(1-2):49-55

95. Blask De, et al. Light during darkness, melatonin suppression and cancer progression. Neruo Endocrino Lett. 2002 Jul;23 Suppl 2:52-6

96. Vijayalaxmi, et al. Melatonin as a radioprotective agent: a review. Int J Radiat Oncol Biol Phys. 2004 Jul 1;59(3):639-53

97. Rodriguez C, et al. regulation antioxidant enzymes: a significant role for melatonin. J Pineal Res. 2004 Jan;36(1):1-9

98. Srinivasan V. Melatonin oxidative stress and neurodegenerative diseases. Indian J Exp Biol. 2002 Jun;40(6):668-79

99. Cuzzocrea S, Reiter RJ. Pharmacological actions of melatonin in acute and chronic inflammation. Curr Top Med Chem. 2002 Feb;2(2):153-65

100. Acuna-Castroviejo D, et al. Mitochondrial regulation by melatonin and its metabolites. Adv Exp Med Biol. 2003;527:549-57

101. Morales AJ, et al. Effects of replacement dose of dehydroepiandrosterone in men and women of advancing age. J Clin Endocrino Metab. 1994 Jun;78(6):1360-7

102. Villareal DT, Holloszy, JO. Effect of DHEA on abdominal fat and insulin action in elderly women and men. JAMA. 2004 Nov 10; 292(18): 2243-48

103. Luo S, et al. Effect of dehydroepiandrosterone on bone mass, serum lipids and dimethylbenz(a)anthracene-induced mammary carcinoma in the rat. Endocrinology. 1997 Aug;138(8):3387-94

104. Green JE, et al. 2-difluoromethylornithine and dehydroepiandrosterone inhibit mammary tumor progression but not mammary or prostate tumor initiation in C3(1)SV40 T/t-antigen transgenic mice. Cancer Res. 2001 Oct 15;61(21):7449-55

105. Couillard S, et al. Effect of dehydroepiandrosterone and the anti-estrogen EM-800 on growth of human ZR-75-1 breast cancer xenografts. J Natl Cancer Inst. 1998 May 20;90(10):772-80

106. Schmitt M, et al. Dehydroepiandrosterone stimulates proliferation and gene expression in MCF-7 cells after conversion to estradiol. Mol Cell Endocrinol. 2001 Feb 28;173(1-2):1-13

107. Johnson, MD, et al. Uses of DHEA in aging and other disease states. Ageing Res Rev. 2002 Feb;1(1):29-41

108. Lissoni P, et al. Dehydroepiandrosterone sulfate secretion in early and advanced solid neoplasms: selective deficiency in metastatic disease. Int J Biol Markers. 1998 Jul-Sep;13(3):154-7

109. Dorgan JF, et al. Relationship of serum dehydroepiandrosterone, DHEA sulfate, and 5-androstene-3 beta, 17 beta-diol to risk of breast cancer in postmenopausal women. Cancer Epidemiol Biomarkers Prev.1997 Mar;6(3):177-81

110. Labrie F, et al. DHEA and its transformation into androgens and estrogens in peripheral target tissues: intracrinology. Front Neuroendocrinol. 2001 Jul;22(3): 185-212

111. Labrie F, et al. Endocrine and intracrine sources of androgens in women: inhibition of breast cancer and other roles of androgens and their precursor dehydroepiandrosterone. Endocr Rev.2003 Apr;24(2):152-82.

112. Stroll BA. Dietary supplements of dehydroepiandrosterone in relation to breast cancer risk. Eur J Clin Nutr. 1999 Oct;53(10):771-5

113. Onland-Moret NC, et al. Urinary endogenous sex hormone levels and the risk of postmenopausal breast cancer. Br J Cancer. 2003 May 6;88(9):1394-9

114. Key TJ, et al. Body mass index, serum sex hormones, and breast

cancer risk in postmenopausal women. J Natl Cancer Inst. 2003 Aug 20;95(16):1218-26

115. Dimitrakakis C, et al. A physiologic role for testosterone in limiting estogenic stimulation of the breast. Menopause. 2003 Jul-Aug;10(4):274-6

116. Ando S, et al. Breast cancer: from estrogen to androgen receptor. Mol Cell Endocrinol. 2002 Jul31;193(1-2):121-8

117. Davidson SL, Davis SR. Androgens in women. J Steroid Biochem Mol Biol. 2003 Jun;85(2-5):363-6

118. Rudman D, et al., Effects of human growth hormone on men over 60 years old. N Eng J Med. 1990 Jul 5;323(1):52-4

119. Besson A, et al., Reduced longevity in untreated patients with isolated growth hormone deficiency. J Clin Endocrinol Metab. 2003 Aug;88(8):3664-7

120. Ruiz-Torres A, Soares de Melo Kirzener M. Ageing and longevity are related to growth hormone/insulin like growth factor-1 secretion. Gerontology 2002 Nov-Dec;48(6):401-7

121. Furstenberger G, Senn HJ. Insulin-like growth factors and cancer. Lancet Oncol. 2002 May;3(5):298-302

122. Stoll BA. Breast cancer: further metabolic-endocrine risk markers? Br J Cancer. 1997;76(12):1652-4

123. Susan E Hankinson, et al. Circulating levels of insulin-like growth factor 1 and risk of breast cancer. Lancet. 1998 May 9;351(9113):1393-6

124. Pratt SE, Pollak MN. Insulin like binding protein 3 (IGFBP-3) inhibits estrogen-stimulated breast cancer cell proliferation. Biochem Biophys Res Commun. 1994 Jan 14;198(1)292-7

125. Madrid O, et al. Growth hormone protects against radiaotherapy-induced cell death. Eur J Endocrinol.2002 Oct;147(4):535-41

126. Crist DM, Kraner JC. Supplemental growth hormone increases the tumor cytotoxicity activity of natural killer cells in healthy adults with normal growth hormone secretion. Metabolism. 1990 Dec;39(12):1320-4

127. Savino W, et al. In vivo effects of growth hormone on thymic cells. Ann NY Acad Sci. 2003 May;992:179-85

128. Khorram O, et al. Effects of growth hormone releasing hormone (GHRH) administration on the immune system of aging men and women. J Clin endocrine Metab. 1997 Nov;82(11):3590-6

129. Serri O, et al. Alteration of monocyte function in patients with growth hormone deficiency: effect of substitutive GH therapy. J clin Endocrine Metab. 1999 Jan;84(1):58-63

130. Cherbonnier C, et al. Potentiation of tumour apoptosis by human

growth hormone via glutathione production and decreased NF-Kappa B activity. B J Cancer, 2003 Sep 15;89(6):1108-15

131. Wright NM, et al. Increased serum 1,25-dihydroxyvitamin D after growth hormone administration is not parathyroid hormone mediated. Calcif Tissue Int. 1997 Aug;61(2):101-3

132. Nam SY, et al. Low dose growth hormone treatment combined with diet restriction decreases insulin resistance by reducing visceral fat and increasing muscle mass in obese type 2 diabetic patients. Int J Obes Relat Metab Disod. 2001 Aug;25(8)1101-7

133. Webb SM, et al. Oncologic complications of excess GH in acromegaly. Pituitary. 2002 Jan;5(1):21-5

134. Smyth PP. The thyroid and breast cancer: a significant association. Ann Med. 1997 Jun;29(3):189-91

135. Strain JJ, et al., Thyroid hormones and selenium status in breast cancer. Nutr Cancer. 1997;27(1):48-52

136. Kmiec Z, et al. Natural Killer cell activity and thyroid hormones in young and elderly persons. Gerontology. 2001 Sep-Oct;47(5):282-8

137. Nakanishi K, et al. Triiodothyronine enhancesw expression of the interleukin-2 receptor alpha chain. Endocr J. 1999 Jun;46(3):437-42

138. Gonzalez-Sancho JM, et al. Inhibition of tenascin-C epression in mammary epithelial cells by thyroid hormone. Mol Carcinog. 1999 Feb;24(2):99-107

139. Gonzalez-Sancho JM, et al. Inhibition of proliferation and expression of T1 and Cyclin D1 genes by thyroid hormones in mammary epithelial cells. Mol Carcinog.2002 May;34(1):164

140. Martinez MB, et al. Altered response to thyroid hormones by prostate and breast cancer cells. Cancer Chemother Pharmacol.2000;45(2):93-102

141. Gregoraszczuk EL, et al. Thyroid hormone inhibits aromatase activity in porcine thecal cells cultured alone and in combination with granulose cells. Thyroid. 1998 Dec;8(12):1157-63

142. Krotkiewski M, et al. Small doses of triiodothyronine can change some risk factors associated with abdominal obesity. Int J obes Relat Metab Disord. 1997 Oct;21(10):922-9

143. Adan RA, et al. Thyroid hormone regulates the oxytocin gene. J Biol Chem 1992 Feb 25;267(6):3771-7

144. Antipenko Aye, Antipenko YN. Thyroid hormones and regulation of cell reliability systems. Adv Enzyme REgul. 1994;34:173-98

145. Cassoni P et al. Oxytocin modulates estrogen receptor alpha expression and function in MCF7 human breast cancer cells. Int J Oncol 2002 Aug;21(2):375-8

146. Cassoni P, et al., Biological relevance of oxytocin and oxytocin receptors in cancer cells and primary tumors. Ann Oncol. 2001;12 Suppl 2:S37-9
147. Chiodera P, et al. Relationship between plasma profiles of oxytocin and adrenocorticortropic hormone during suckling or breast stimulation in women. Horm Res 1991;35(3-4):119-23
148. Mezzacappa ES, Katlin ES. Breast-feeding is associated with reduced perceived stress and negative mood in mothers. Health Psychol. 2002 Mar;21(2)187-93
149. Wihko RK, Apter DL. The epidemiology and endocrinology of the menarche in relation to breast cancer. Cancer Surv. 1986;5(3):561-71
150. Moore JW, et al. Sex hormone binding globulin and breast cancer risk. Anticancer Res. 1987 Sep-Oct;7(5B):1039-47
151. Bulbrook RD, et al. Sex hormone binding protein and the natural history of breast cancer. ANN N Y Acad Sci. 1988;538:248-56
152. Fortunati N, et al. Sex hormone binding globulin, its membrane receptor, and breast cancer: a new approach to the modulation of estradiol action in neoplastic cells. J Steroid Biochem Mol Biol. 1999 Apr-Jun:69(1-6):473-9
153. fortunati N. Sex hormone binding globulin: not only a transport protein. What news is around the corner? J Endocrinol Invest. 1999 Mar;22(3):223-34
154. Pugeat M, et al. Clinical utility of sex hormone binding globulin measurement. Horm Res. 1996;45(3-5):148-55
155. Krotkiewski M, et al. Small doses of triiodothyronine can change some risk factors associated with abdominal obesity. Int J Obes Relat Metab Disord. 1997 Oct:21(10):922-9
156. Bauman AE. Updating the evidence that physical activity is good for health: an epidemiological review 2000-2003. J Sci Med Sport. 2004 Apr;7(1Supppl):6-19
157. Lee IM. Physical activity and cancer prevention-data from epidemiologic studies. Med Sci Sports Exerc; 2003Nov;35(11):1823-7
158. Thune I, et al. Physical activity and the risk of breast cancer. N Eng J Med. 1997 May 1;336(18):1269-75
159. Thune I, Furberg AS. Physical activity and cancer risk, all sites and site specific. Med Sci Sports Exerc. 2001 Jun;33(6 Suppl):S530-50
160. Lagerros YT, et al. Physical activity in adolescence and young adulthood and breast cancer risk: a quantitative review. Eur J Cancer Prev. 2004 Feb;13(1):5-12
161. Bruce CR, Hawley JA. Improvement in insulin resistance with aerobic exercise training: a lipocentric approach. Med Sci Sports Exerc. 2004 Jul;36(7):1196-201

162. Ross R. et al. Exercise-induced reduction in obesity and insulin resistance in women: a randomized controlled trial. Obes Res. 2004 May;12(5):789-98

163. McTiernan A, et al; Effect of exercise on serum estrogens in postmenopausal women: a 12 month randomized clinical trial. Cancer Res. 2004 Apr 15;64(8)2923-8

164. Tymchuk CN, et al. Changes in sex hormone binding globulin, insulin and serum lipids in post menopausal women on a low fat high fiber diet combined with exercise. Nutr Cancer. 2000;38(2):158-62

165. Kraemer WJ, et al. The effects of short-term resistance training on endocrine function in men and women. Eur J Appl Physiol Occup Physiol. 1998 Jun; 78(1):69-76

166. Raastad T, et al. Hormonal responses to high and moderate intensity strength exercise. Eur J Appl Physiol. 2000 May;82(1-2):121-8

167. Hurel SJ, et al. Relationship of physical exercise and ageing to growth hormone production. Clin Endocrinol (Oxf).1999 Dec;51(6):687-91

168. Nemet D, et al. Negative energy balance plays a major role in the IGF-1 response to exercise training. J Appl Physiol. 2004 Jan;96(1):276-82

169. Schmitz KH, et al. Effects of a 9-month training intervention on insulin, insulin like growth factor (IGF-1) IGF-binding protein 1 and IGFBP3 in 30 to 50 year old women. Cancer Epidemiol Biomarkers Prev. 2002 Dec;11(12):1597-604

170. Djuric Z, et al. Oxidative DNA damage levels in blood from women at high risk for breast cancer are associated with dietary intakes of meats, vegetables and fruits. J AM Diet Assoc. 1998 May;98(5):524-8

171. Ingram DM, et al. Effect of low fat diet on female sex hormone levels. Natl Cancer Inst. 1987 Dec;79(6):1225-9

172. Welsch CW. Relaltionship between dietary fat and experimental mammary tumorigenesis: a review and critique. Cancer Res 1992 Apr 1; 52(7 Suppl):2040-48

173. Lee MM, Lin SS. Dietary fat and breast cancer. Annu Rev Nutr. 2000;20:221-48

174. Shin MH, et al. Intake of dairy products, calcium, and vitamin D and risk of breast cancer. J Natl Cancer Inst. 2002 Sep 4;94(17):1301-11

175. Lipworth L, et al. Olive oil and human cancer: an assessment of the evidence. Prev Med. 1997 Mar-Apr;26(2):181-90

176. Trichopoulou A, Lagiou P. Worldwide patterns of dietary lipids intake and health implications. Am J Clin Nutr. 1997 Oct;66(4 Suppl):961S-64S

177. Trichopoulou A, et al. Cancer and Mediterranean dietary

traditions. Cancer Epidemiol Biomarkers Prev. 2000 Sep;9(9):869-73

178. Moral R, et al. Modulation of EGFR and new expression by n-6 and n-9 fat diets in experimental mammary adenocarcinomas. Oncol Rep. 2003 Sep-Oct;10(5):1417-24

179. Terry PD, et al. Intakes of fish and marine fatty acids and the risks of cancers of the breast and prostate and of other hormone related cancers: a review of the epidemiologic evidence. Am J Clin Nutr. 2003 Mar;77(3):532-43

180. Stoll BA. N-3 fatty acids and lipid peroxidation in breast cancer inhibition. Br J Nutr. 2002 Mar;87(3):193-8

181. Smith-Warner SA, et al. Intake of fruits and vegetables and risk of breast cancer: a pooled analysis of cohort studies. JAMA. 2001 Geb 14;285(6):799-801

182. Hung T, et al. Fat Versus carbohydrate in insulin resistance, obesity, diabetes and cardiovascular disease. Curr Opin Clin Nutr Metab Care. 2003 Mar;6(2):165-76

183. Rock Cl, et al. Effects of high-fiber, low-fat diet intervention on serum concentration of reproductive steroid hormones in women with a history of breas cancer. J Clin Oncol. 2004 Jun 15;22(12)2379-87

184. Fowke JH, et al. Brassica vegetable consumption shifts estrogen metabolism in healthy postmenopausal women. Cancer Epidemiol Biomarkers Prev. 2000 Aug;9(8):773-9

185. Xa X. et al. Soy consumtion alters endogenous estrogen metabolism in postmenopausal women . Cancer Epidemiol Biomarkers Prev.2000 Aug;9(8):781-6

186. La Vecchia C, et al. Vegetables, fruits, anti-oxidants and breast cancer: a review of Italian studies. Eur J Nutr. 2001 Dec;40(6):261-7

187. Sato R, et al. Prospective study of carotenoids, tocopherols, and retinoid concentrations and risk of breast cancer. Cancer Epidemiol Biomarkers Prev. 2002 May;11(5):451-7

188. Dorgan JF, et al. Relationships of serum carotenoids, retinol, alph-tocopherol, and selenium with breast cancer risk: results from a prospective study in Columbia, Missouri (United States). Cancer Causes Control. 1998 Jan;9(1):89-97

189. Zhang SM. Role of vitamins in the risk, preventon and treatment of breast cancer. Curr Opin Obstet Gynecol. 2004 Feb;16(1):19-25

190. Kline K, et al. Vitamin E and breast cancer prevention: current status and future potential. J Mammary Gland Biol Neoplasia. 2003 Jan;8(1)91-102

191. Jiang Q, et al. Gamma-tocopherol, the major form of vitmin E in the US diet, deserves more attention. Am J Clin Nutr. 2001 Dec;74(6):714-22

192. Hensley K, et al. New perspectives on vitamin E: gamma-tocopherol and carboxyelthylhydroxychroman metabolites in biology and medicine. Free Radic Biol Med. 2004 Jan 1;36(1):1-15
193. Kim YI. Folate and cancer prevention: a new medical application of folate beyond hyperhomocysteinemia and neural tube defects. Nutr Rev. 1999 Oct;57(10):314-21
194. Zhang S, et al. A prospective study of folate intake and the risk of breast cancer. JAMA. 1999 May 5'281(17):1632-7
195. Prinz-Langenohl R, et al. Beneficial role for folate in the prevention of colorectal and breast cancer. Eur J Nutr. 2001;40(3):98-105
196. Choi Sw. Vitamin B 12 deficiency: a new risk factor for breast cancer. Nutr Rev.1999 Aug;57(8):250-3
197. Vieth R. Vitamin D supplementation, 25-hydroxyvitamin D concentrations, and saftety. Am J Clin Nutr. 1999 May;69(5):842-56
198. Holick MF. Vitamin D: A millennium perspective. J Cell Biochem. 2003 feb 1;88(2):296-307
199. Calvo MS, Whiting SJ. Prevalence of vitamin D insufficiency in Canada and United States: importance to health status and efficacy of current food fortification and dietary supplement use. Nutr Rev. 2003 Mar;61(3):107-13
200. Kurtzke JF, et al. Epidemiology of multiple sclerosis in U.S. veterans: Race, sex and geographical distribution. Neurology, 1979 Sep;29(9 Pt 1):1228-35
201. Ponsonby AL, et al. Ultraviolet radiation and autoimmune disease: insights from epidemiological research. Toxicology. 2002 Dec 27;181-182:71-8
202. Nieves J, et al. High prevalence of vitamin D deficiency and reduced bone mass in multiple sclerosis. Neurology. 1994 Sep;44(9):1687-92
203. Li YC Vitamin D regulation of the resin-angiotensin system. J Cell Biochem. 2003 Feb 1;88(2):327-31.
204. Hanchette CL, Schwartz GG. Geographic patterns of prostate cancer mortality. Evidence for a protective effect of ultraviolet radiation. Cancer. 1992 Dec 15;70(12):2861-9
205. Garland CF, et al. Calcium and vitamin D; their potential roles in colon and breast cancer prevention. Ann N Y Acad Sci. 1999:889:107-19
206. Welsh J, et al. Vitamin D-3 receptor as a target for breast cancer prevention. J Nutr. 2003 Jul;133(7 Suppl):2425S-2433 S
207. Lowe L, et al. Mechanisms implicated in the growth regulatory effects of vitamin D compounds in breast cancer cells. Recent Results Cancer Res. 2003;164:99-110

208. Guyton KZ, et al. Vitamin D and vitamin D analogs as cancer chemopreventive agents. Nutr Rev. 2003 Jul;61(7):227-38

209. OKelly J, Koeffler HP. Vitamin d analogs and breast cancer. Recent results Cancer Res. 2003;164: 333-48

210. Vinceti M, et al. The epidemiology of selenium and human cancer. Tumori. 2000 Mar-Apr;86(2):105-18

211. El-Bayoumy K, Sinha R. Mechanisms of mammary cancer chemoprevention by organoselenium compounds. Mutat Res. 2004 Jul 13;551(1-2):181-97

212. Medina D, et al. Se-methylselenocysteine: a new compound for chemoprevention of breast cancer. Nutr Cancer. 2001;40(1):12-7

213. Kellis JT Jr, Vickery LE. Inhinition of human estrogen sythetase (aromatase) by flavones. Science. 1984 Sep 7;225(4666):1032-4

214. Jeong HJ, et al. Inhibition of aromatase activity by flavonoids. Arch Pharm Res. 1999 Jun;22(3):309-12

215. Campbell DR, Kurzer MS. Flavonoid inhibition of aromatase enzyme activity in human pre adipcytes. J Steroid Biochem Mol Biol. 1993 Sep;46(3):381-8

216. Kodama N, et al. Effects of D-fraction, a polysaccharide from Grifola frondosa on tumor growth involve activation NK cells. Biol Pharm Bull. 2002 Dec;25(12):1647-50

217. Kodama N, et al. Effect of Maitake (Grifola frondosa) D-Fraction on the acrtivation of NK cells in cancer patients. J Med Food. 2003 Winter;6(4):371-7

218. Kodama N, et al. Can maitake MD-fraction aid cancer patients? Altern Med Rev. 2002 Jun;7(6):236-9

219. Yagita A, et al. H-2 haplotype-dependent serum IL-12 production tumor-bearing mice treated with various mycelial extracts. In Vovo, 2002 Jan-Feb;16(1):49-54

220. Matsui Y, et al. Improved prognosis of postoperative hetocellular carcinoma patients when treated with functional foods; a prospective cohort study. J Hepatol. 2002 Jul;37(1):147-50

221. Levy J, et al. Lycopene is a more potent inhibitor of human cancer cell proliferation than either alpha carotene or beta carotene. Nutr Cancer. 1995;24(3):257-67

222. Karas M, et al. Lycopene interferes with cell cycle progression and insulin-like growth factor 1 signaling in mammary cancer cells. Nutr Cancer;2000;36(1)101-11

223. Chalabi N, et al. The effects of lycopene on the proliferation of human breast cells and BRCA1 and BRFCA2 gene expression. Eur J Cancer. 2004 Jul;401(11):1768-75

224. Nahum A, et al. Lycopene inhibition of cell cycle progression in

breast and endometrial cancer cells is associated withreduction in cyclin D levels and retention of p27 in the cycin E-cdk2 complexes. Oncogene. 2001 Jun 7;20(26):3428-36

225. La Veechia C. Tomatoes, lycopene intake, and digestive and female hormone-related neoplasms. Exp Biol Med (Maywood). 2002 Nov;227(10):860-3

226. Terry P, et al. Dietary carotenoids and risk of breast cancer. Am J Clin Nutr. 2002 Oct;76(4):883-8

227. Hulten K, et al. Carotenoids, alpha-tocopherols, and retinol in plasma and breast cancer risk in northern Sweden. Cancer Causes Control. 2001 Aug;12(6):529-37

228. Sato R, et al. Prospective study of carotenoids, tocopherols and retinoid concentrations and the risk of breast cancer. Cancer Epidemiol Biomarkers Prev. 2002 May;11(5):451-

229. Bradlow HL, et al. Multifunctional aspects of the action of indole-3-carbinol as an anti-tumor agent. Ann N Y Acad Sci. 1999;889:204-13

230. Rahman KM, et al. Indole-3-carbinol induces apoptosis in tumorigenic but not in nontumorigenic breast epithelial cells. Nutr Cancer. 2003;45(1):1010-12

231. Rahman KM, et al. Inactivation of akt and NF-kappa B play important roles during indole-3-carbinol-induced apottosis in breast cancer cells. Nutr Cancer. 2004;48(1):84-94

232. Meng Q et al. Suppression of breast cancer invasion and migration by indole 3 carbinol: associated with upregulation of BRCA! And E-cadherin/catenin complexes. J Mol Med 2000;78(3):155-65

233. Meng Q, et al. Inhibitory effects of Indole-3-carbinol on invasion and migration in human breast cancer cells. Breast Cancer Res Treat. 2000 Sep;63(2):147-52

234. Meng Q, et al. Indole-3-carbinol is a negative regulator of estrogen receptor-alpha signaling in human tumor cells. J Jutr. 2000 Dec;130(12):2927-31.

235. Lee I J, et al. Inhibition of MUCI expression by indole-3-carbinol. Int J Cancer. 2004 May 10;109(6):810-6

236. Chatterji U, et al. Indole-3-carbinol stimulates transcription of the interferon gamma receptor 1 gene and augments interferon reponsiveness in human breast cancer cell. Carcinogenesis. 2004 Jul;25(7):1119-28

237. Bradlow HL, et al. Long-term responses of women to indole-3-carbinol or a high biber diet. Cancer Epidemiol Biomarkers Prev. 1994 Ont-Nov;3(7):591-5

238. Wong GY, et al. Dose-ranging study of indole-3-carbinol for

breast cancer prevention. J Cell Biochem Suppl. 1997;28-29:111-6

239. Kitani K, et al. Interventions in aging and age associated pathologies by means of nutritional approaches. Ann N Y Acad Sci. 2001 Jun:1019:424-6.

240. Komori A, et al. anticarcinogenic activity of green tea polyphenols. Jpn J Clin Oncol. 1993 Jun;23(3):186-90

241. Satoh K, et al. Inhibition of aromatase activity by green tea extract catechins and their endocrinological effects of oral administration in rats. Food Chem Toxicol. 2002 Jul;40(7):925-33

242. Mittal A, et al. EGCG down-regulates telemetase in human breast carcinoma MCF-7 cells, leading to suppression of cell viability and induction of apoptosis. Int J Oncol. 2004 Mar;24(3):703-10

243. Masuda M, et al. Epigallocatechin-3-gallate inhibits activation HER-2/neu and downstream signaling pathways in human head and neck and breast carcinoma cells. Clin Cancer Res. 2003 Aug 15;9(9):3486-91

244. Yeh CW, et al. Suppression of fatty acid synthase in MCF-7 breast cancer cells b tea and tea polyphenols: a possible mechanism for their hyplipidemic effects. Pharmacogenomics J. 2003;3(5):267-76

245. Sartippour MR, et al. Inhibition of fibroblast growth factors by green tea. Int J Oncol. 2002 Sep;21(3):487-91

246. Sartippour MR et al. Green tea inhibits vascular endothelial growth factor (VEGF) induction in human breast cancer cells. J Jutr. 2002 Aug;132(8):2307-11

247. Liberto M, Cforbrinik D. Growth factor-dependent induction p21 by green tea polypheno, epigallocatechin gallate. Cancer Lett. 2000 Jun 30;154(2):151-61

248. Suzuki Y, et al. Green tea and the risk of breast cancer: pooled analysis of 2 studies in Japan. Br J Cancer. 2004 Apr 5;90(7):1361-3

249. Nakachi K, et al. Can teatime increase one's lifetime? Ageing Res Rev. 2003 Jan;2(1):1-10

250. Sartippour MR, et al. Green Tea and its catechins inhibit breast cancer xenografts. Nutr Cancer . 2001;40(2):149-56

251. Kavanagh KT, et al. Green tea extracts decrease carcinogen-induced mammary tumor burnden in r4ats and rate of breast cancer cell pliliferation in culture. J Cell Biochem. 2001;82(3):387-98

252. Nakachi K, et al. Influence of drinking green tea on breast cancer malignancy among Japanese patients. Jpn J Cancer Res. 1998 Mar;89(3):254-61

253. Inoue M, et al. Regular consmtion of green tea and the risk of breast cancer recurrence: follow-up study from the hospital-based epidemiologic research program at Aichi Cancer Center (HERPACC), Japan. Cancer Lett. 2001 Jun 26;167(2):175-82

254. Wu AH, et al. Green tea and risk of breast cancer in Asian Americans. In J Cancer.2003 Sep 10;106(4):574-9

255. Fujiki H, et al.Mechanistic findings of green tea as cancer preventive for humans. Proc Soc Exp Bio Med. 1999 Apr;220(4):225-8

256. Guastalla JP, et al. Cyclooxygenase 2 and breast cancer, From biological concepts to therapeutic trials. Bull Cancer. 2004 May;91 Spec No:S99-108

257. Denkert C, et al. Prognostic impact of cyclooxygenase-2 in breast cancer. Clin Breast Cancer. 2004 Feb;4(6):428-33

258. Bosetti C, et al. Aspirin and cancer risk: an update to 2001. Eur J Cancer Prev. 2002 Dec;11(6):535-42

259. Moran EM. Epidemiological and clinical aspects of nonsteroidal anti-inflammatory drugs and cancer risks. J Environ athol Toxicol Oncol. 2002;21(2):193-201

260. Wang D, Dubois RN. Cyclooxygenase-2: a potential target in breast cancer. Semin Oncol.2004 feb;31(1 Suppl3):64-73

261. Chow LW, et al. Celeecoxib anti-aromatase neoadjuvant (CAAN) trial for locally advanced breast cancer: preliminary report. J Steroid Biochem Mol Biol. 2003 Sep;86(3-5):443-7

262. Arun B, Goss P. The role of COX-2 inhibition in breast cancer treatment and prevention. Semin Oncol. 2004 Apr;31(2 Suppl 7):22-9

263. Bleiker EM, van der Ploeg HM. Psychosocial factors in the etiology of breast cancer: review of a popular link. Patient Educ Couns. 1999Jul:37(3):201-14

264. Dalton SO, et al. Mind and cancer. Do psychological factors cause cancer? Eur J Cancer. 2002 Jul;38(10):1313-23

265. Reiche EM, et al. Stress, depression, immune system, and cancer. Lancet Oncol. 2004 Oct;5(10):617-25

266. Montazeri A, et al. The role of depression in the development of breast cancer: analysis of registry data from a single institute. Asian Pac J Cancer Prev. 2004 Jul-Sep;5(3)316-9

267. Jacobs JR, Bovasso GB. Early and chronic stress and their relation to breast cancer. Psychol Med. 2000 May;30(3):669-78